Bart Depreitere

Spinal Surgery

for Physiotherapists

Lannoo
Campus

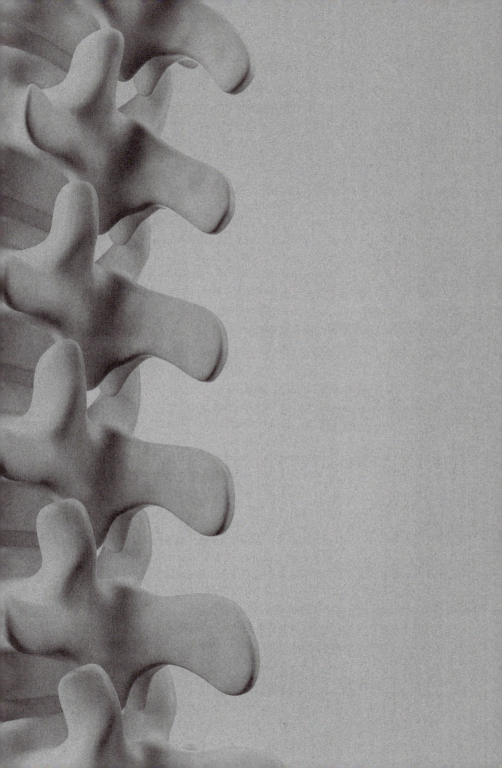

CONTENTS

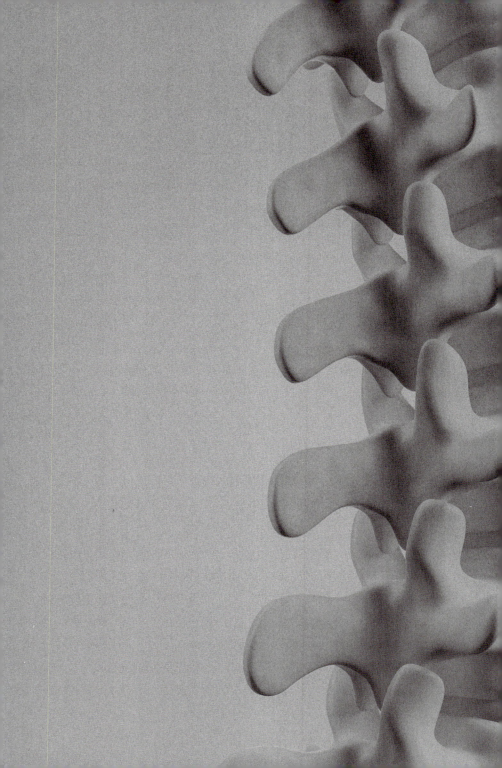

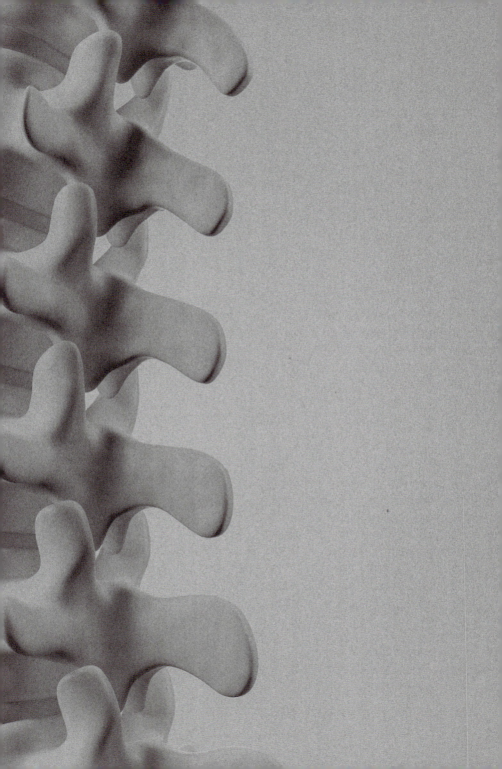

PREFACE

It may seem weird to write a book on surgery for non-surgeons. Yet, it is not. In the surgical management of spinal problems, three things are extremely important. The first (and possibly most crucial) element is the correct indication for surgery. In many (degenerative) cases, the indication depends, among others, on the nature and quality of conservative therapy being offered to the patient before surgery is even considered. Hence, as the physiotherapist and rehabilitation physician are inevitably part of a multidisciplinary team, they should at least be aware of the exact role of surgery, and know what surgery can and cannot achieve. Second, when a decision in favour of surgery has been made, preoperative optimisation of the patient's condition, management of expectations and fears, perioperative guidance and postoperative management are of utmost importance. The latter includes the optimisation of coping, the optimisation of soft tissue healing, the management of misbalance and dysfunction and the gradual training towards activities and participation based on needs and wishes. These objectives can be obtained through a combination of education and psychosocial guidance, exercises, manual therapy, ergonomic advice and psychomotor therapy, chosen and customised to the individual patient. In fact, postoperative physiotherapy does not necessarily differ from conservative therapy, but the therapist should be aware of the particularities and potential consequences of the surgery. Finally, when individual experts of different disciplines speak a common language and give the same messages to the patient during the entire pre-, peri- and postoperative process, a reassuring cloud of trust and positivism will surround the patient and the team and will reinforce the teamwork to achieve a good outcome in all aspects. Where knowledge, skills and empathy have always been essential to any professional caregiver, multidisciplinarity – and, even better, interdisciplinarity – has become an indispensable virtue.

This little book is subdivided into chapters per spinal region, and covers most relevant pathologies for each region. At the end, it contains a vocabulary of surgical procedures, which aims at improving the understanding of surgical terminology and appropriate communication among caregivers and with patients. The book is intended for all physiotherapists and rehabilitation physicians dealing with spinal problems. In addition, it serves as course text for the spinal surgery section of the truncus *Selected topics in musculoskeletal pathology'* in KU Leuven's 2nd master physiotherapy curriculum. This course brings medical specialist knowhow to the physiotherapist and aims at bridging the challenging gap between medical reasoning and the functional objectives associated with the International Classification of Functioning, Disability and Health. Teaching young physiotherapists with one foot in medical practice and one in rehabilitation pushes the medical specialist out of his comfort zone and forces him to summarise his background knowledge and experience into clear, comprehensive and consistent concepts. Therefore, this book may bring a view that is somewhat more generic than usual, original and maybe thought-provoking. For the latter reason and because medical literature is a very dynamic field, I deliberately did not include literature references, although I assure the reader that the insights provided are based on common evidence and in line with existing guidelines.

I sincerely hope this work can help the course participants, and physiotherapists and rehabilitation physicians outside the course, to better understand surgical reasoning in spinal pathologies and thereby cross the bridge somewhat more than halfway, because it is there that sparks may produce a wonderful fire that enlightens the entire field.

Bart Depreitere

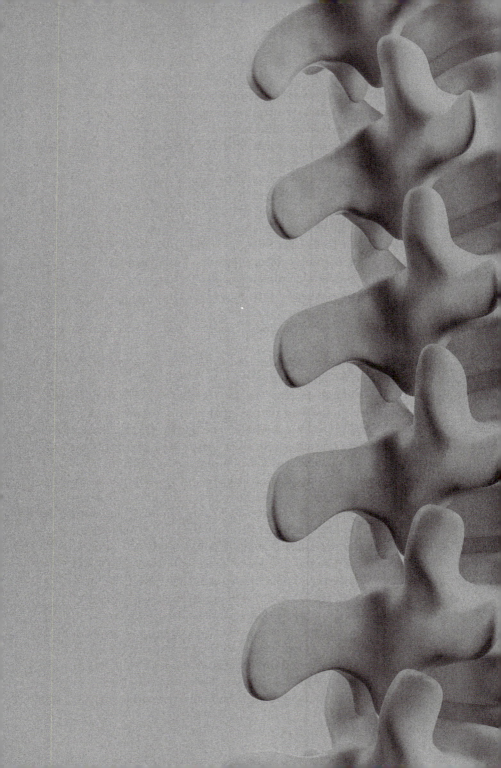

Knowledge is not something you own.
It is a gift you should relish, nourish,
make tastier, or more abundant
to pass it on to the next generation
in the interest of humanity.
If you hide it, you kill it.

Bart Depreitere

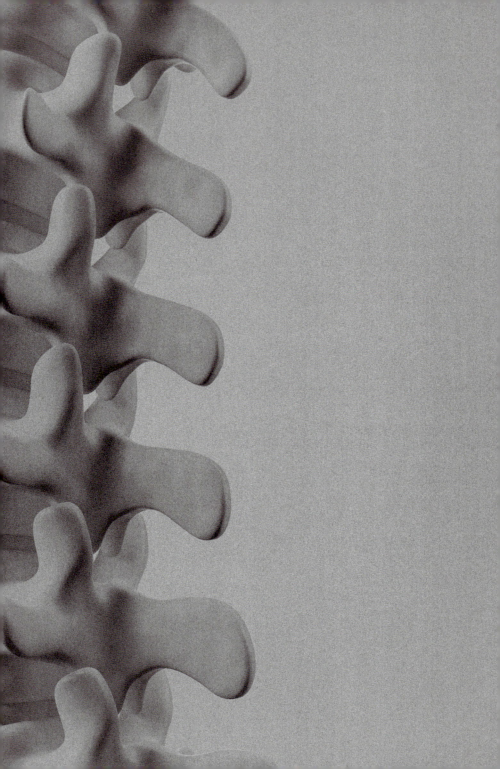

INTRODUCTION

HISTORY AND CURRENT CONCEPTS ON THE ROLE OF SURGERY IN SPINAL MANAGEMENT

NUMBER ONE CAUSE OF DISABILITY

Worldwide, low back pain is the number one cause of years lived with disability. This is only different in regions with war or natural disasters, and in the United States, where opioid addiction supersedes any other condition. The lifetime prevalence of low back pain is over 80%, meaning that almost every adult will be confronted with at least one episode of low back pain during his or her life. This should not necessarily surprise us, since our spine was originally not designed to be in an upward position for most of the day. The first historical note on low back pain was found in ancient Egypt, shortly after the introduction of writing. Therefore, it is reasonable to state that low back pain is part of our human condition; a flaw just like greed and envy.

So, why does back pain receive so much medical attention, if it has been part of life since ancient history – probably long before and certainly thereafter? In 1862, *The Lancet* issued its first report on 'The Influence of Railway Travelling on Public Health'. With the advent of organised labour in an industrialised context – the railway workers being one of the first groups in whom this became apparent – back pain became a phenomenon that could not simply be ignored anymore, as it affected work capacity. In the centuries before, back pain was considered a form of rheumatism, and some early schools in the eighteenth and nineteenth century advocated exercise, while others promoted rest. Now, back pain had become a societal problem, never to disappear. Social legislation, including workers compensation introduced after World War II, inadvertently made the problem a lot larger. Some authors therefore consider low back disability a product of industrial society. Of note, the problem is not confined to the decreasing number of workers performing hard manual labour, but affects the entire working community.

Meanwhile, medical science has made progress. Roentgen images were introduced in the late nineteenth century. For the first time, people could associate pain with image findings, and not surprisingly, surgeons started to believe that the lumbosacral anomalies discovered on the imaging were the cause of back pain. However, attempts to intervene failed. History repeated itself when magnetic resonance imaging (MRI) was introduced in the nineties. Now, the world of soft tissues could be assessed. And black discs (discs somewhat degenerated in terms of hydration content) were believed to be the main culprit. Since at the same time spinal osteosynthesis hardware became commercialised, a tremendous wave of arthrodesis surgeries overwhelmed Western countries, and failed again. The biopsychosocial model, introduced by Waddell in 1987, appeared to be much closer to the truth than initially admitted. It is now recognised that psychosocial risk factors explain a large part of outcome variability after treatment. Anyhow, the damage was done: modern medicine made back pain a disease.

HISTORY OF SPINAL SURGERY

It is heartwarming that the first lumbar disc surgery in 1934 was performed by a neurosurgeon (Mixter) together with an orthopaedic surgeon (Barr). What was formerly believed to be a chondroid tumour causing sciatica turned out to be a piece of normal disc extruding from the disc space representing a totally benign degenerative condition. Verbiest, a Dutch neurosurgeon, discovered lumbar spinal canal stenosis to be the cause of neurogenic claudication (Verbiest's syndrome) in 1954, and proposed surgical laminectomy as treatment. Spinal arthrodesis development had a truly orthopaedic origin. Bone fusions using pieces of rib after removal of sick vertebral bodies became a successful surgical treatment for the often devastating Pott's disease (spinal tuberculosis). Hence, it was proven that bone fusion in the spine was feasible. On a different note, Harrington in the United States and Cotrel and Dubousset in France started to become successful in correcting severe malaligned curvatures in adolescent idiopathic scoliosis, thereby introducing the first metal hardware as a means of reduction and internal fixation. It consisted of rods and frames on the one hand, and wire and hooks on the other hand to fasten to the spine. Now it was only necessary to bring the hardware and bone fusion concepts from the pioneers together to create a story of greater success.

In 1973, Roy-Camille, a Parisian orthopaedic surgeon, introduced the pedicle screws for the lumbar spine and lateral mass screws in the cervical spine, setting the stage for shorter and more versatile constructs, and for surgical solutions in many more spinal conditions. Industry took over from here and was the real driving force for any later technical novelty: cages to replace discs and facilitate fusion, transmuscular minimal access technology, and most recently, endoscopy. Surgeons needed these innovations to further push the boundaries, eg. in deformity corrections, en bloc tumour removal, transnasal endoscopic odontoid surgery and other complex and challenging spinal pathologies.

CURRENT CONCEPTS ON THE ROLE OF SURGERY IN SPINAL MANAGEMENT

We should be well aware that the role of surgery in the management of spinal problems is rather limited. Surgery can play a role in a vast number of disorders, but when taking into account the overwhelming prevalence of axial pain problems in which surgery has little to no contribution, only a small proportion of patients are potential beneficiaries. Surgical help may be required in red flag pathologies and persistent radicular pain, however not in the large majority of neck and back pain problems that reflect a mechanical overload to a system with insufficient load bearing capacity. On the contrary, surgery in such cases may have a negative effect on pain, dysfunction and their spontaneous evolution when poorly applied, and it may be counterproductive in terms of the patient's attitudes and beliefs. Therefore, surgery may eventually contribute to poor outcomes, called 'failed back management syndrome' (AKA failed back surgery syndrome).

The triage system that is acknowledged in many international guidelines, and that was reinforced in the Belgian national low back pain pathway developed by the Health Knowledge Centre (KCE) and the Spine Society of Belgium in collaboration with all relevant stakeholders, offers the best possible guidance for case management. First, we screen for red flags. Red flags are indicators of potentially harmful conditions if not well recognised and treated, such as fever, weight loss, oncological history, sudden deformity, preceding trauma, etc. They have a rather moderate individual sensitivity, but when considered in clusters of meaningful stories (traumatic injury, tumour, infection ...) the sensitivity rises significantly. In case of suspicion of a red flag situation, patients should be swiftly referred for further imaging (in an emergency or within days depending on the situation) and when confirmed, will end up in a specific pathway that may well include surgery (see further in this book).

Once red flags are ruled out, we look for radicular pain, with its characteristic findings (pattern of radiating pain, provocable radiating pain, and possible associated neurological symptoms). In radicular pain, strength should be checked since considerable (< 4/5 on the MRC scale) recent (no more than a couple of days) loss of strength may be an indication for urgent surgical decompression, and hence, should be referred accordingly. If strength is accurate, the timeline comes into effect: acute (< 6 weeks) radicular pain should not be operated on because chances of spontaneous improvement are huge. Injections can be considered when pain is too intense while waiting. In the subacute stage, several options are possible: painkillers while awaiting natural improvement, additional physiotherapy, injections and surgical decompression. In chronic radicular pain, a surgical consultation is advocated in all patients in order to facilitate proper and well-informed shared decision making. Surgery may consist of pure decompression, but in some instances, more elaborate procedures (including arthrodesis) may be required. Psychosocial risk factors may play a role in decision making and consideration to include additional coaching and closer guidance of the patient.

Once radicular pain is ruled out, we arrive in the group of axial pain, again with a timeline. In the acute stage, emphasis is on reassurance, comfort and activation. From 2 weeks onwards, checking the risk factors for unfavourable outcome or chronification is advisable (STarT Back, Örebro) and patients with high risk factors should be offered physiotherapy. In subacute axial pain, efforts should be increased in order to avoid chronicity, titrating efforts based on the evolution of the discomfort and on the presence of risk factors. Inclusion in interdisciplinary rehabilitation programmes under the supervision of specialists in physical medicine may be required. In chronic low back pain, rehabilitation potential and risk factors should be carefully studied in order to direct patients to the best suited management pathways. Many patients with unused rehabilitation potential and low to moderate risk factors should be managed under the guidance of physical medicine specialists. Patients with low rehabilitation potential and/ or considerable risk factors are better off in pain clinics focusing on symptoms and support. There are some very selective indications for surgery in axial pain (see later in this book) under the condition that the rehabilitation potential is studied first and that the physical medicine specialists agree that surgery is the better option before proceeding to renewed rehabilitation.

The role of surgeons and surgery, as well as the role of any medical specialty and management modality, in pain and dysfunction of lumbar origin is very nicely outlined in the Belgian pathway (see www.lowbackpain.kce.be), and similar principles can be applied in cervical and thoracic spinal problems.

THE FUTURE

We are not at the end stage of our capacity to understand and manage spinal problems. If we were, low back pain would not be the number 1 cause of years lived with disability. Tackling this astonishing truth should become a major objective. Building further on the knowledge and experience collected in the previous decades, we need to build a uniform multiaxial diagnostic framework for patients with axial pain and invest in the refinement and standardisation of diagnostic criteria, rehabilitation and surgical management elements as well as outcome measures in order to facilitate accurate comparison of study results and enable large(r) meta-analyses. Finally, we should establish large prospective multicentre data repositories for comparative effectiveness research that should allow us to identify treatments that work better than others. The tools and instruments exist for advanced data processing; now it is up to us to build high quality databases. In parallel, fundamental lab research on degeneration may deliver clues for actual repair. Ideally, initiatives are governed internationally, because if we all keep doing our own little research, we will never reach the big objective. A challenging future is ahead of us.

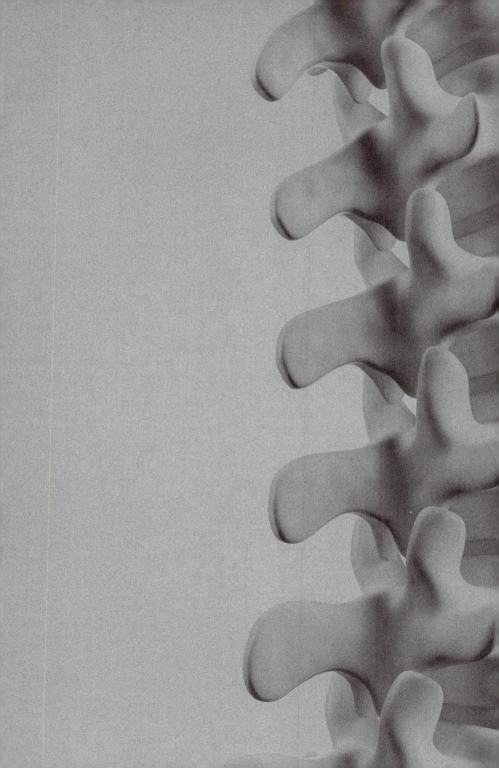

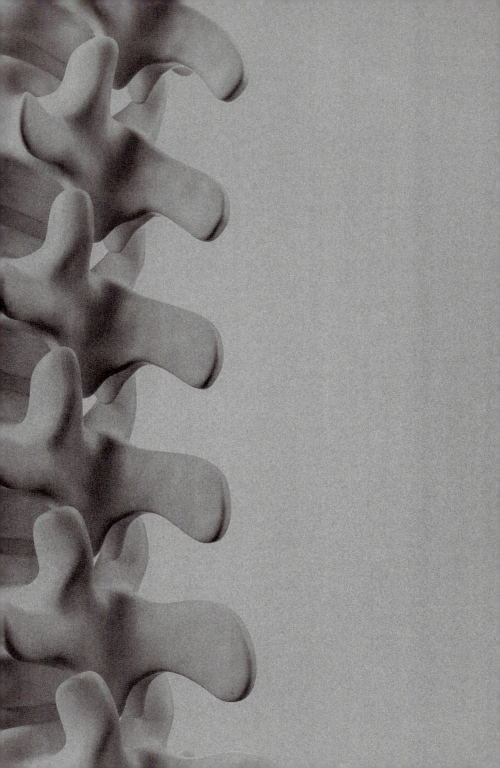

PART 1

A SURGICAL PERSPECTIVE ON THE CERVICAL SPINE

1. SURGICAL APPROACHES TO THE CERVICAL SPINE

The cervical spine can be surgically approached from the anterior (ventral) or posterior (dorsal). In the anterior approach, an oblique or horizontal incision is made along the medial border of the sterno-cleidomastoid muscle. Next, by further dissection medial to the neurovascular bundle and lateral to the thyroid gland, the anterior cervical spine can easily be reached by gently pushing the trachea and oesophagus away from the midline. On the anterior cervical spine, we see the two longus colli muscles, which have to be dissected away to have a sufficiently wide access. This manoeuvre allows one to expose the spine from the inferior edge of C2 to the superior edge of T1 and sometimes even T2. This anterior approach is elegant because it uses natural planes between these structures and causes almost no postoperative pain. When the approach is slightly modified to go lateral to the neurovascular bundle, the lateral edge of the transverse process is reached, giving access to the lateral cervical spine. To approach the anterior arch of C1, the odontoid, the body of C2 and the clivus, a route via the mouth and opening the midline raphe of the oropharynx muscle, or transoral approach, can be performed. Alternatively and more often performed nowadays, one can use the transnasal endoscopic approach to the anterior upper cervical spine.

From the posterior side, by making a midline incision and dissecting the avascular plane of the ligamentum nuchae onto the spinous processes and further between the muscles and bones, one can expose the laminae and lateral masses C2-C7 (and further down), posterior arch of C1 and occipital bone. Sometimes, the surgeon will choose a transmuscular approach by making a more lateral incision, and dividing the fascia and muscles to arrive at the junction between the laminae and the lateral masses, eg. when using transmuscular tubes for a foraminotomy.

The muscle manipulation associated with the posterior approach causes postoperative pain, which is much less the case in the anterior approach. The anterior approach however can cause temporary dysphagia (as a result of manipulation of the oesophagus) and hoarseness (recurrent laryngeal nerve). The transoral route requires nil per os for several days until the pharynx mucosa has healed, which is less problematic in the transnasal approach. The posterior approach allows for decompression techniques, such as foraminotomy, laminectomy and laminoplasty, that do not create instability and therefore do not require arthrodesis. In the ventral approach, decompression implies a discectomy or corpectomy, which should always be followed by reconstruction and arthrodesis. When removing the odontoid complex, ligamentous instability is the result and a posterior occipitocervical arthrodesis needs to follow.

So, what can a surgeon achieve in the cervical spine? Apart from reducing tumour or infection load, one can achieve decompression of the spinal cord, nerve roots or a vertebral artery (the latter indication is rare). Depending on the approach, this should be accompanied by arthrodesis, which will usually imply osteosynthesis as well as bone fusion. In trauma surgery or situations of instability, stabilisation without decompression can be indicated. In the cervical spine, this will also usually involve osteosynthesis as well as bone fusion. Next, extensive surgery can be performed to correct severe cervical deformities. Artificial discs or disc prostheses have been developed for the cervical spine – their objective being to maintain motion in young patients after anterior discectomy, not to restore motion. However, it has been demonstrated that this motion is non-physiological and not superior to classic arthrodesis. Restoring motion, unfortunately, is not possible to date. At best, one can try to avoid arthrodesis in order to preserve motion by choosing a decompression technique that does not require subsequent arthrodesis.

2. TRAUMA OF THE CERVICAL SPINE

Cervical spine injuries are frequent, particularly in poly-trauma patients that were the victims of a high energy trauma and in head injured patients. Due to its high range of motion, the cervical spine is prone to injury: about one third of all spinal injuries occur in the cervical spine. Because these injuries are frequent and because there is a risk of spinal cord injury in undiagnosed cervical trauma, the cervical spine should be immobilised at the scene of any accident and be formally 'cleared' by a spine surgeon at the emergency department. This is done by history taking and clinical examination, and by imaging that is performed whenever there is the least level of suspicion. Most injuries involve bone fractures, but ligamentous injuries should not be overlooked. Of course, combinations of both may also occur. Fragments can be displaced or non-displaced. CT-scanning is the imaging modality of choice, its sensitivity being much higher than X-ray. For all high energy traumas and for all traumas requiring CT-scanning of other body regions, a CT-scan of the cervical spine should be preferred over X-rays for the assessment of cervical injuries. One should be aware, however, that the CT-scan is a static examination and is not able to visualise ligamentous injury. When ligamentous injury is suspected, MRI is the preferred modality.

In general, lesions that compromise the stability of the cervical spine and hence threaten the spinal cord should be stabilised surgically. Lesions that are considered 'stable' can heal with immobilisation. Unfortunately, no consensus definition exists on what is considered stable and what is not. For bone fractures, assessment of stability depends on parameters such as type, location and extent of the fracture within the Dennis 3-column concept (anterior, middle and posterior column), vertebral body height loss, kyphotic angulation and fracture comminution. Ligamentous injuries usually do not heal spontaneously and often require surgical stabilisation. Finally, cord compression by disrupted bone fragments or cervical spine displacement (luxation) requires decompression or reduction, and subsequent stabilisation. Reduction can be obtained through gradual traction, manual reduction or open (surgical) reduction. Surgical stabilisation is obtained by surgically introducing osteosynthesis hardware. Immobilisation of the cervical spine can be obtained in a hard collar or by applying a halo-jacket. A soft-collar is by no means a form of immobilisation.

Immobilisation is usually adequate in the following injuries:
- Most occipital condyle fractures
- After successful reduction of a C1C2 rotatory subluxation without transverse ligament rupture
- Most Jefferson fractures (C1 ring fractures)
- Type 3 odontoid fractures (fracture through the base of the odontoid in the C2 body)
- Some Hangman fractures (C2 bilateral pedicle fracture)
- Lamina and spinous process fractures
- Most unilateral lateral mass fractures in the subaxial (C3-C7) cervical spine
- Most subaxial (C3-C7) body compression fractures (compression fracture only concerns the anterior column)

Surgical stabilisation in the cervical spine will usually consist of both osteosynthesis and bone fusion, and is warranted in:
- Occipitocervical arthrodesis in craniocervical dislocation (complete ligamentous rupture between the skull and C1/C2)
- C1C2 arthrodesis in transverse ligament rupture, C1C2 rotatory

subluxation impossible to reduce and type 2 odontoid fracture (fracture through the mid-part of the odontoid). In the latter case, an odontoid screw may also be placed.

- ACIF in most Hangman fracture types (C2 bilateral pedicle fracture), subaxial facet fracture luxations, subaxial bilateral lateral mass fractures, subaxial ligamentous failure
- Corpectomy and anterior arthrodesis in most subaxial burst fractures (burst fracture involves the anterior and middle column)
- Posterior cervical arthrodesis as an adjunct to anterior constructs or as a single construct in ligamentous injuries.

In Whiplash grades 1, 2 and 3, surgery is not required and patients should get appropriate education by a physiotherapist, who supports soft tissue healing and advises on posture and motion, to gradually switch to exercises when deemed necessary. If patients do not get better soon, they should be referred to a physical medicine specialist for more elaborate rehabilitation, well before the pain becomes chronic, and ideally after a couple of weeks.

Cervical spine injuries account for half of spinal cord injuries. After resuscitation and immobilisation, patients are brought to the emergency department, where a complete neurological exam and swift imaging are performed. More and more evidence advocates urgent surgery for decompression of the spinal cord and subsequent stabilisation. Patients with a cervical spinal cord injury are prone to respiratory problems, because they usually lose at least part of their intercostal muscle function, which is needed for deep breathing and coughing when being recumbent (be aware that in addition, these patients are often being operated on and temporarily intubated, after which they have to rely on their adjunct respiratory muscles even more). Patients with impaired diaphragm function in high cervical cord lesions are dependent on mechanical ventilation. Also, blood pressure should be kept high enough to ensure sufficient spinal cord perfusion. For these reasons, and to avoid and monitor for other complications such as thrombo-embolism, gastroparesis and ileus, urinary tract infections, etc., these patients belong in the intensive care ward for at least a couple of days. Neuro-rehabilitation should be started soon, and is currently already initiated in the acute phase at the intensive care. Besides motor and (gnostic and vital) sensory deficits, sphincter control and autonomous function can be impaired, the latter manifesting itself in deficient temperature control and sudden blood pressure drops. Gradually, hypertonia and spasticity associated with upper motor neuron injury will occur.

3. CERVICAL RADICULAR PAIN

Most radicular conditions have nerve root compression in their etiology. The mechanical compression does certainly play a significant role in the pathogenesis of pain and associated symptoms. However, it does not explain the entire picture. Radicular symptoms may resolve spontaneously, while on imaging the structures causing compression are still there. It is largely assumed that inflammatory processes, such as the release of cytokines, are responsible for or at least associated with the generation of radicular symptoms. These inflammatory processes may gradually calm down, explaining spontaneous resolution of symptoms. The degenerative causes of radicular compression are usually located at the very proximal part of the nerve root, where it branches off the spinal cord and enters the foramen. The compression may be caused by a disc herniation or an osteophyte, and most often it is the combination of both at the same time. A pure soft disc herniation is composed of nucleus pulposus and is secondary to weakening of the annulus fibrosus. Its location can vary from median to lateral. The paramedian position, i.e. right off the midline, is most frequent. The origin of osteophytes is most often from the uncovertebral joint and compress the nerve root inside the foramen. Osteophytes may also arise from the endplates or the facet joint. Rarely, nerve root compression is caused by non-degenerative pathologies, such as an epidural abscess or a tumour.

The predominant symptom caused by nerve root irritation in the cervical spine is radicular arm pain, which can be intense and debilitating. The onset of the radicular pain may be very sudden, sometimes after a certain movement or activity, but can also be gradual over days or weeks. Radicular pain has 3 main characteristics. First, the pain follows some kind of a pattern in its downwards course in the arm. In many instances this pattern matches more or less with the corresponding dermatome of the irritated nerve root. In degenerative conditions of the cervical spine, the nerve roots that are most frequently involved are C6 and C7; less often, C5 and C8. Although the pain pattern may be difficult to describe for patients, some patients will be able to tell that, as an example, the pain goes all the way to their thumb in a C6 root problem. Be aware, however, that this is not always so confined and overlap between dermatomes may occur.

Second, radicular pain can be provoked. Typically, when a disc herniation causes the nerve root compression, Valsalva manoeuvres (sneezing, coughing) will provoke arm pain. If a foraminal stenosis causes the nerve root compression, the pain may be provoked by extension of the neck (which may however also be the case in a discogenic problem). The hyperextension-compression test and the Spurling test can be used as provocative tests for radicular arm pain. Third, radicular pain can be associated with neurological symptoms (the so-called 'radiculopathy'). Patients may complain of tingling and/or hypoesthesia (loss of sensation) in the involved dermatome. Moreover, muscle weakness can occur in the myotome associated with the involved nerve root. A decrease in or absence of muscle reflexes can be associated: biceps and brachioradialis reflex for C6 and triceps reflex for C7. Finally, neck pain can be associated but is a variable and non-specific symptom.

When trying to differentiate between degenerative radicular pain and other causes of arm pain, one should discriminate between three main entities: radicular pain, peripheral neuropathy and musculoskeletal disorders. Typical of radicular pain is the pattern and the potential association of the pain with neurological signs and symptoms (see above) more or less confined to dermatomes and myotomes. Typical of compressive radicular pain is that the pain can be provoked by Valsalva manoeuvres and by irritative tests such as Spurling.

Degenerative conditions are the most frequent cause of compressive radicular pain. However, compression may also result from mass lesions such as tumours or abscesses. Often, red flags (weight loss, fever, pain at night ...) will be present in that case, which is the reason why red flags should be screened for at each contact. Finally, not all radicular conditions are caused by compression. Parsonage-Turner syndrome is an inflammatory idiopathic condition of the brachial plexus; it is characterised by severe arm and shoulder pain and weakness in the arm. Typically more than one nerve root is involved in the clinical picture. This, together with the severe pain at the onset, should be the clue to think of this condition. Herpes zoster infections may represent another cause of dermatome-related pain.

Peripheral neuropathies such as carpal tunnel syndrome and cubital ulnar nerve compression are relatively frequent causes of tingling and hypoesthesia in the fingers and may be associated with muscle weakness and pain. In carpal tunnel syndrome, tingling will typically be present at night, when the hand is not moving and venous congestion increases. The tingling is confined to the thumb and index (and sometimes third finger) and radial side of the hand, where hypoesthesia may also be present. Muscle weakness, if present, will include the thumb opposition, and the thenar may be hypotrophic. Patients will mention that shaking the hand diminishes the tingling. Pain may be present in the forearm and thumb/index. Only rarely does the pain go higher than the elbow. The Tinel test, which provokes the tingling by tapping on the nerve, can be positive at the flexor ligament at the wrist. The most frequent location of ulnar nerve compression is in the cubital tunnel at the medial epicondyle of the elbow. Tingling appears in the 4th and 5th digit and is typically provoked by elbow flexion or leaning on the elbow. Hypoesthesia may be associated. Weakness will include finger adduction and little finger abduction. The hypothenar may be hypotrophic. Relief of tingling may be obtained by stretching the elbow. The Tinel test can be positive at the cubital tunnel.

Polyneuropathy is caused by vascular damage to the finest endings of nerves. This can result from diabetes, renal failure, chemotherapy, or inflammatory conditions. Typically the longest nerves (hands and foot) are affected first. Patients will complain of numbness and tingling in the hands, and usually also in the feet, with the so-called 'glove and sock' distribution.

The most frequent musculoskeletal disorders that are confused with cervical radicular pain are the impingement syndromes in the shoulder. These will often cause pain that is, however, typically confined to the upper arm. One should not forget that shoulder and cervical spine degeneration may occur simultaneously and hence, both may contribute to arm pain to a certain extent. Typically, pain will be provoked by abduction and endo- or exorotation in the shoulder. In addition, referred pain in the arm may arise from muscular or articular origin in the neck, eg. first rib dysfunction, and is usually called pseudoradicular pain.

When acute (less than 6 weeks) radicular pain is suspected and red flags are ruled out, management is conservative, unless the radicular pain is complicated by significant weakness or in the rare case when the pain is really unbearable in spite of accurate medical management. This means that at each contact, strength should be examined. Strength deficits existing for less than a couple of days are amenable to emergency surgical decompression, which improves strength prognosis. Although there is no good evidence, this is probably similar to lumbar radicular weakness, in which it has been demonstrated that less than 4/5 on the MRC is alarming, while for 4/5 or better there is clinical equipoise on whether surgery or conservative therapy works best. It is probably best to refer each patient with acute loss of strength for emergency surgical advice. Whatever therapy is chosen, muscle strength exercising will be a helpful adjunct.

In acute radicular pain without strength deficit, initial therapy is conservative because of significant chances of spontaneous improvement, i.e. without surgical intervention. Conservative therapy will consist of reassurance, explaining the suspected problem and emphasising the positive natural evolution in the large majority of patients, comfort measures including painkillers and the advice to remain as active as possible. When psychosocial risk factors are present, closer follow up and coaching is recommended, and these patients, eg. with counteractive emotions, kinesophobia or catastrophising beliefs, are better off under the guidance of a physiotherapist for education and psychosocial guidance. Graded exercises may be useful to help the patient back to the premorbid status, while the role of specific physiotherapy actions is still unclear. Imaging is not recommended, as it will not change management. Again, emphasis is on the spontaneous natural resolution and every action should be taken to facilitate this. When the pain is too intense, an injection of steroids under fluoroscopic guidance in a pain clinic can be an option in order to obtain more effective temporary pain relief. In the latter case, imaging will be required to pinpoint the area of compression and to guide the subsequent infiltration.

In the subacute stage (6-12 weeks), the above options are still valid, but also surgery can be an option in a shared decision making setting. Therefore, it is very useful that the physiotherapist is aware of the nature, goals, risks and circumstances of surgery to properly advise patients of all possible options. If the pain has neuropathic characteristics (burning sensation, allodynia, hyperalgia, sensation of warmth or cold), the patient should be referred to a physician for specific treatment with atypical painkillers (eg. amitriptyline, gabapentin, pregabalin ...). In the chronic stage (12 weeks and longer) a surgery consult is strongly advisable. This does not mean that the patient should necessarily be operated on, but the patient is entitled to a surgical expert opinion on what surgery is about to obtain faster pain relief.

The main goal of surgery in cervical radicular pain is to relieve the radicular pain in the arm. Significant reduction of radicular pain is achieved immediately or shortly after surgery in over 90 percent of patients provided the diagnosis and indication were correct. The effect of surgery on neck pain is very unpredictable and neck pain itself is usually a poor indication for any surgical action. Surgery may improve chances of recovery of muscle weakness if performed within hours (to a couple of days maximum) of the onset of weakness. Finally, loss of sensation only recovers very slowly and gradually, with or without surgery, and therefore hypoesthesia on its own is a poor indication for surgery.

In theory, surgery can be performed from the front or from the back. Anterior surgery consists of a complete discectomy, after which the source of compression can be removed. Following this manoeuvre, a reconstruction of the removed intervertebral disc is required. In the original technique described by Cloward in the 1950s (Mulier and

Dereymaeker from Leuven described this technique at the same time
at a Parisian congress) this was done by introducing an iliac crest bone
autograft. Nowadays, surgeons will usually introduce a PEEK, carbon or titanium cage filled with bone or bone substitute in between
the endplates (anterior cervical interbody fusion, ACIF). In order to
achieve immediate stability, a thin plate can be screwed onto the anterior walls of the above and below vertebral bodies, taking care not to
get too near to the adjacent disc levels, since the overarching of a plate
over a mobile disc will promote adjacent level degeneration.

Even when properly performed, the lever arm of two vertebrae including a fused disc will execute increased loading forces and pressure in
the adjacent discs, which will accelerate degenerative changes (adjacent
level degeneration). It has been demonstrated that about one third of patients develop adjacent level degeneration over the following 10 years,
and 10 percent of them become symptomatic (the latter being called adjacent level disease). In order to prevent the phenomenon of adjacent
level degeneration and disease, the cervical artificial disc was invented
and first human implantation occurred in Leuven in 2000. The artificial
discs do allow the index segment to remain mobile and do decrease the
rate of adjacent level degeneration, but only to a very limited extent that
is clinically irrelevant and does not justify its high cost. Therefore, cervical artificial discs have largely been abandoned.

Posterior surgery consists of making an approach in between the upper
and lower lamina by resecting the yellow ligament and then removing a
small medial part of the facet joint to expose the exiting nerve root. By
mobilising the nerve root, the disc herniation or osteophyte anterior to
it can be approached through the shoulder or armpit of the nerve root.
The huge advantage of such posterior surgery is the avoidance of a fusion and its associated long-term risk for adjacent level disease. Also,
when the incision and muscle manipulation are kept minimal, it is possible to perform this surgery with minimal neck pain (neck pain being a
downside of posterior surgery). However, it is the exact location and nature of the compression that will determine whether or not a posterior
surgery is at all possible. This is because it is immensely important not
to manipulate the spinal cord. As a result, the posterior approach is only

indicated in situations of lateral nerve root compression, i.e. lateral to the thecal sac. A herniated lateral disc sequester can easily be removed by mobilising the nerve root, but the limited space makes it difficult and potentially dangerous to drill out osteophytes from posteriorly. Therefore, the posterior approach, usually referred to as foraminotomy, will only be used for the surgical management of lateral (i.e. intraforaminal) disc herniations, while all other problems (paramedian disc herniation, any osteophytic problem) will be tackled through anterior decompression and ACIF. In all surgical procedures, optical magnification is applied by means of loupes or (preferably) a microscope.

ACIF is a frequently performed surgery with minimal risks. About one third of the patients has a postoperative dysphagia that usually resolves over weeks. Some patients develop hoarseness, which is usually also temporary, unless the recurrent laryngeal nerve is injured. An oesophageal breach may lead to mediastinitis and is a life-threatening complication that is fortunately really rare. Vertebral artery injuries have also rarely been described, which is also the case for spinal cord injuries (<1%). The main risk is in applying an inappropriate technique that may lead to non-union and/or hardware failure, and associated neck pain. Postoperative infection risk is less than 1%. For the foraminotomy procedure, nerve root or spinal cord injury and postoperative wound infection have been reported, but again the chances are very low (<1%).

Whatever approach and procedure is chosen, the patient is allowed to mobilise the neck immediately after the surgery. Neck pain is seen more often in posterior surgeries than in ACIF surgery, although the distraction during discectomy and cage introduction may irritate the facet joints and result in postoperative interscapular pain. The benefit of postoperative physiotherapy has not been formally proven. However, why should one prove the obvious? Patients will have questions and worries and a postoperative physiotherapy consult at the ward is an absolute minimum. This therapist can decide whether or not further postoperative sessions at home seem advisable to reinforce education and help the patient to be fit for work and regain participation after 4 to 6 weeks. Physiotherapy is usually beneficial in this phase, as little as possible but as much as needed.

4. CERVICAL DEGENERATIVE MYELOPATHY[1]

The normal sagittal diameter of the subaxial spinal canal is 14-22 mm. There is enough space for the spinal cord and the roots, the ligaments, veins and epidural fat. Degenerative changes of the cervical spine can cause a slow and gradual narrowing of the cervical spinal canal and may lead to spinal cord compression. Anatomical substrates that contribute to the narrowing are the disc (disc protrusions, disc bulging), the endplates (osteophytes), the posterior longitudinal ligament (degenerative thickening or ossification of the ligament), the facet joint (osteophytes and hypertrophy) and the yellow ligament (degenerative disorganisation and hypertrophy of the ligament). Additional narrowing may be caused by degenerative anterolisthesis or retrolisthesis and by compensatory hypermobility usually at levels cranial to degenerative ankylotic levels.

Spinal cord compression may be asymptomatic when it is mild. Studies have shown that long tract signs are occurring when the cross-sectional area of the cord is reduced by 30% or more. Apart from static narrowing, dynamic factors also play a role. In flexion, the cord may be stretched over osteophytic spurs of the endplates. More importantly, in extension the canal diameter narrows further due to buckling of the yellow ligament. At the tissue level, compression and its associated potential dynamic worsening leads to mechanical cord injury. Moreover, it has been shown that blood supply may become compromised, adding to the injury. The end-result of both is demyelination. Apparently, the corticospinal tracts are particularly vulnerable to this process.

Degenerative cervical myelopathy, i.e. myelopathy secondary to degenerative cervical spinal canal stenosis compressing the spinal cord, is usually characterised by a slow and gradual onset of symptoms. Typically, initial subtle symptoms include clumsiness and numbness/ tingling of the hands along with gait instability and urinary urge or urge incontinence. The clumsiness of the hands results from discrete

---

1   myelopathy = pathologic condition of the spinal cord (myelon)
(≠ myopathy: pathological condition of the muscles)

functional damage to the corticospinal tracts. The gait instability is due to impaired function of the posterior funiculi, which carry proprioceptive information. The urinary urge results from functional damage to the inhibitory spinal cord tracts that impair bladder emptying when it is full (parasympathetic loop). In this early stage, clinical examination may reveal a positive Romberg test, i.e. unsteadiness when standing upright with the legs together and the eyes closed due to impaired proprioception. Tendon reflexes may be vivid. Hoffmann's test is usually positive as well, as a result of upper motor neuron impairment. If Hoffmann's is negative, it may become positive in neck extension due to additional narrowing of the canal in extension. Some patients will report a sensation of electricity going down over the trunk in neck flexion. This phenomenon is called Lhermitte's phenomenon.

When the disease is progressive, long tract signs will become more apparent and include spasms and spastic gait. Gait ataxia will result from worsening of proprioceptive dysfunction and eventually ambulation will become impossible. At the same time, areflexia, hypoesthesia and neuropathic burning pain may develop in the arms due to nerve root entry zone compression.

The natural evolution of the disease tends to progression. However, this progression is generally slow to very slow, with two thirds of patients remaining stable over the course of several years in published series. Sometimes, progression is more stepwise with intermittent periods of quiescence. Occasionally, however, the development of clinical myelopathy may be subacute and ambulation may be lost over the course of weeks. Patients with moderate to severe symptoms and functional decline, and certainly patients with clear progression, are candidates for surgical decompression. In patients with only mild symptoms and little functional consequences, the current strategy is to offer close clinical follow up (whereas in the past those patients were usually operated on). Of note, hyperextension trauma in cervical spinal stenosis may cause contusions of the spinal cord (i.e. central cord syndrome) that can result in devastating neurological deficits, ranging from tetraplegia to distal upper limb weakness. However, the low frequency of this condition does not justify preventive surgery in stenosis patients. Only if a patient is prone to falling, prevention of additional traumatic sequelae might be an additional argument pro surgical decompression.

As outlined above and as has been demonstrated in literature, patients with moderate to severe myelopathy are better off with surgical decompression to arrest the progression of the disease. The severity of the functional impact of the disease is easily determined by applying the internationally recommended mJOA (modified Japanese Orthopaedic Association) score. Postoperatively, the majority of patients do improve in terms of neurological function, although this cannot be guaranteed nor predicted with current diagnostic tools. In other words, the goal of surgery is to stop potential further deterioration and offer a reasonable chance for improvement while at the same time avoiding neurological complications from the surgery. In patients with mild myelopathy and in whom no surgery is offered while following up on the patient, it may be useful in some cases to offer neurological physiotherapy to improve or maintain hand function and gait at the best possible level.

As in cervical radicular pain, surgical decompression can be obtained from the front or from the back. Anterior techniques include discectomy and ACIF, exactly the same technique as for radicular pain in which this time the protruding disc and/or endplate osteophytes causing anterior spinal cord compression are removed, and corpectomy. In a corpectomy, except for the lateral walls and transverse processes the entire vertebral body is resected in a piecemeal fashion, including the disc above and below. This is performed when anterior spinal cord compression is mainly present at body level, and in this case it is usually caused by thickening of the posterior longitudinal ligament. Following corpectomy, a reconstruction is achieved by the introduction of a cage of sufficient height, again filled with autologous bone or bone substitute, and always finished off by a plate and screws.

Posterior techniques include laminectomy, laminectomy and arthrodesis, and laminoplasty. Laminectomy, the removal of an entire lamina, including its spinous process and the yellow ligament above and below it, and being performed at one or multiple levels, is without doubt the oldest technique. A laminectomy at multiple levels is definitely effective, but associated with a certain percentage of long-term secondary neurological deterioration – probably due to the cervical muscles adhering directly onto the thecal sac and potentially causing repetitive spinal cord irritation during muscle contraction – and a certain percentage of postoperative progressive kyphosis and neck pain – due to the loss of the posterior tension band. The American school advocates to have all laminectomies associated with posterior arthrodesis, which is done by screws in the lateral masses and which provides better long-term outcomes. The latter is true, but more aggressive, and for mono- or bisegmental compression a single level laminectomy is probably in the grey area where neither one nor the other is superior. Skip laminectomy is a relatively new and promising technique, in which much attention is paid to sparing of muscle attachments and in which not all but alternating laminae are removed.

In a laminoplasty or 'open door laminoplasty', the cervical lamina is cut at one side and thinned on the other side, and then opened to the side of the thinning, which acts as a hinge by creating a greenstick fracture. On the other side, the lamina is kept open by a small piece of metal or bone. This technique offers the advantage of installing a barrier between the thecal sac and muscles and mobility is maintained. It is associated with a certain percentage of long-term postoperative kyphosis, but without this being associated with neurological worsening. Relatively similar outcomes have been described in laminectomy with arthrodesis and in laminoplasty. In fact, trials and retrospective series that investigated the superiority of the anterior versus posterior techniques could not find significant differences either. The latter is likely explained by the immense heterogeneity of the anatomical characteristics in terms of number of levels, exact causes of compression and cervical alignment. This is exactly what surgeons look at to decide what type of surgery they will perform: 1) does the compression on the cord mainly come from an anterior or posterior direction?; 2) is the alignment of the cervical spine lordotic or kyphotic?; 3) how many levels are involved? The more kyphotic the spine, the more the surgeon will have to switch to anterior techniques, and the more levels are involved, the less hardware complications are expected from a posterior approach.

Risks of anterior surgery have been described in the chapter on cervical radicular pain, and are the same for discectomy and corpectomy: dysphagia, hoarseness, oesophageal breach (the risk is a bit higher if more levels are involved), vertebral artery injury, spinal cord injury, infection and hardware failure. While the first two are usually temporary side effects, the risk for the other complications is really low, except for hardware failure that increases to being substantial if 3 or more levels are involved in the construction. Since in posterior surgery the thecal sac may be largely exposed, there is a risk for inadvertent spinal cord injury, although in general this is still quite low (<1%). Postoperative neurological decline after spinal cord decompression can occur and rates are variable in literature, but this is usually a temporary phenomenon. Both anterior and posterior surgeries for degenerative myelopathy are associated with a risk of approximately 1% for dural tears and cerebrospinal fluid leakage (5% in revision surgery and 12% in ossified posterior longitudinal ligament). Long anterior and posterior arthrodesis constructs often lead to hypertrophy of the long neck muscles and associated muscular neck pain, due to the functional elimination of the short segment muscles. Finally, both anterior and posterior surgeries carry an average 6% risk for postoperative C5 palsy, probably due to shifting the position of the spinal cord and subsequent traction injury on one or both C5 nerve roots (most horizontal and most prone to traction injury).

The rehabilitation of a patient operated on for cervical degenerative myelopathy is on the edge between musculoskeletal rehabilitation and neuro-rehabilitation, as these patients present with both. Usually, immediately after the surgery, the patient is allowed to mobilise and should not wear a collar. Avoidance of fears, kinesiophobia or over-achieving and guidance on graded activity represent the musculoskeletal aspects. Most often, patients also benefit from gait and agility training. Severely affected patients should be included in (reimbursement) programmes that allow for sufficient intensity and duration of physiotherapy.

5. OTHER THAN TRAUMATIC AND DEGENERATIVE CONDITIONS

The conditions described in this chapter are red flag conditions, most of them being rather rare. The physiotherapist should be able to detect and refer such conditions (see chapter 8), but obviously the patient's trajectory does not stop there. Red flag situations may lead to surgery and require postoperative physiotherapy.

Whereas until the early 2000s spinal metastases were considered an indication for radiotherapy and not for surgery, their prognosis in terms of functional decline and associated withdrawal of onco-logical treatment with subsequent decease was very grim. In 2005 a randomised trial demonstrated that for spinal metastases originating from solid tumours and compressing the spinal cord, the outcome in terms of function, quality of life and survival was much better after surgical debulking and stabilisation followed by radiotherapy than by radiotherapy alone. This landmark trial led to a significant change in management. When patients have a sufficient estimated survival and suffer from a pathological fracture with instability or neurolog-ical worsening from spinal cord compression, a decision for surgery can be taken. Surgery consists of an anterior or posterior approach with tumour debulking and spinal reconstruction. For primary malig-nant bone tumours in the cervical spine, complete resection may be achieved in the context of a multidisciplinary management plan, and those patients should be referred to a specialist tertiary centre.

Infections can occur postoperatively, but the majority of infections encountered in the spine occur without previous spinal surgery and result from haematogenous spread. Indications for surgery are: 1) in-stability from severe osteolysis; 2) spinal cord decompression in case of epidural abscess causing neurological deficits; and 3) severe sepsis not responding to antibiotics and requiring surgical resection of the infection source. The techniques described above (ACIF, corpectomy, laminectomy, laminectomy and arthrodesis) will be applied. Follow-ing accurate debridement and under targeted antibiotics, instrumen-tation hardware can be safely used, even in infection cases.

Inflammatory disorders such as rheumatoid arthritis and Grisel's syndrome, metabolic disorders such as the mucopolysaccharide storage diseases, and congenital disorders such as (complex) Chiari malformations, Klippel-Feil, Down's syndrome and os odontoideum (which may likely be due to a neonatal infection or trauma), mainly affect the craniocervical junction. Instability, either due to ligamentous laxity or a combination of bone malformations and insufficiency, may lead to narrowing of the high cervical canal and high cervical cord compression. In such cases, reduction or decompression along with C1C2 arthrodesis or occipitocervical arthrodesis may be required. In Down's syndrome and achondroplasia, subaxial spinal cord compression, as in degenerative cervical myelopathy, may occur. In patients with ankylosing spondylitis, severe osteoporosis along with spontaneous fusion will result in a brittle bamboo spine. When these patients have neck pain after even a minor trauma, they have a fracture until otherwise proven. These fractures are usually unstable and lead to progressive deformity.

6. POSTOPERATIVE REHABILITATION

The best evidence to date on postoperative rehabilitation in cervical spinal surgery is a recent Swedish randomised controlled trial on 202 postoperative patients that were randomised to either structured postoperative rehabilitation or pragmatic standard approach. No difference in outcome could be detected up to two years of follow up. The study inevitably points at the methodological difficulties associated with investigating effects of physiotherapy, that is per definition individualised and customised. In that regard, it is positive to learn that a randomised trial on 'timeliness incentive nursing', in which patients are effectively encouraged to activate their subjective initiative, did result in faster and better recovery results. There should be no refrain from activation and at least a couple of postoperative physiotherapy contacts are useful to counsel and coach the patient and accommodate his worries, beliefs and practical questions.

A next question is when cervical muscle exercising becomes possible in the postoperative period. Usually, a short period of soft tissue healing will be taken into account before giving the green light. In fact, this green light will usually depend on logistic issues (the first post-operative surgery consult where permission is given may only take place after 6 weeks or longer) and surgeons' beliefs (the bone should be fully healed not to have physiotherapy preclude bone fusion) rather than on rational arguments. The latter argument on bone healing is an interesting one. Reliable bone fusion takes as long as three months or longer. However, not all cervical spine surgeries include bone fusion, eg. laminoplasty or foraminotomy. Also, even if bone fusion is attempted, the use of instrumentation hardware renders the surgical construct sufficiently stable from the start. This means that ACIF without plate and fractures that are immobilised in a collar or halo-jacket are the situations where the physiotherapist should be careful and act in agreement with the surgical follow up. In some of these situations it may be helpful to start conditioning exercises of neck stabilisers and posture towards the end of the bone healing period. Also, gradually tapering immobilisation in stable fractures, eg. moving from a halo-jacket to a collar which is then gradually left off may be useful to account for muscle fatigue. Overall, muscle trauma and need for physiotherapy is usually higher in posterior surgeries.

7. WHAT ABOUT AXIAL PAIN?

Soon after Cloward and his contemporaries developed the ACIF procedure, some surgeons attempted its use in the treatment of axial neck pain without radicular pain and without myelopathy. Many of the reports from those series have serious methodological shortcomings. Studies in which pre- and postoperative change could be reasonably assessed reported only a minority of patients getting better and a substantial proportion not improving or reporting worsening. Guidelines nowadays do not advise the use of surgery in axial neck pain. The answer on how these patients should be addressed is found in the overall triage concept outlined in the introduction of this book.

Red flags should be ruled out first, then radicular pain should be looked for and the management of axial pain depends on the timeline:

the further a patient proceeds in time, the more should be invested in addressing psychosocial risk factors and in avoiding chronicity. In chronic neck pain, rehabilitation potential and all relevant risk factors should be carefully assessed, and in my opinion specialists in physical medicine are in the best position to do this. As stated, surgery should in principle not be performed. However, in medicine, nothing is black or white. Very rarely and after interdisciplinary consultation, surgery may be considered in very selective problems, eg. in severe osteoarthritis of the C1C2 joints.

8. RED FLAGS IN THE CERVICAL SPINE

The below table summarises the cervical red flags, indicators of potentially harmful situations if not recognised. The sensitivity of red flags increases substantially when they are considered in clusters, i.e. in a meaningful story of a suspicious disorder, as outlined below.

CERVICAL MYELOPATHY	• Gait instability, atactic or spastic gait • Disturbed fine motor skills • Urinary urge or urge incontinence • Positive Hoffmann's sign and positive Romberg test • Limb hyperreflexia, pathological cutaneous reflexes, Babinski signs, hypertonia and spastic para- or tetraparesis
INFECTIOUS DISORDER	• Severe and continuous neck pain • Pain worse at night, pain that is not affected by position or movement • Fever, chills • Recent gastro-intestinal/gynaecological infection or surgery • Recent cervical spine surgery • Immune suppression • Intravenous drug use • Recent bacterial infection • Older age

MENINGITIS OR SUBARACHNOID HAEMORRHAGE	• Continuous neck pain (and headache), not position- or movement-related • Meningeal irritation tests positive (neck stiffness, positive Kernig and Brudzinski)
TRAUMATIC FRACTURE OR INSTABILITY	• Possibility of traumatic event • New onset structural spinal deformity • Known or suspected ankylosing spondylitis or DISH and onset of neck pain following (even minor) trauma (= fracture until otherwise proven) • Known or suspected rheumatoid arthritis or metabolic disorder
SPINAL TUMOUR	• New onset neck pain in a patient older than 50 years (55 years in some guidelines) or younger than 20 years • History of cancer • Persistent pain, pain worse at night, pain that is not affected by position or movement • New onset structural spinal deformity • Pain in different locations • Unexplained weight loss

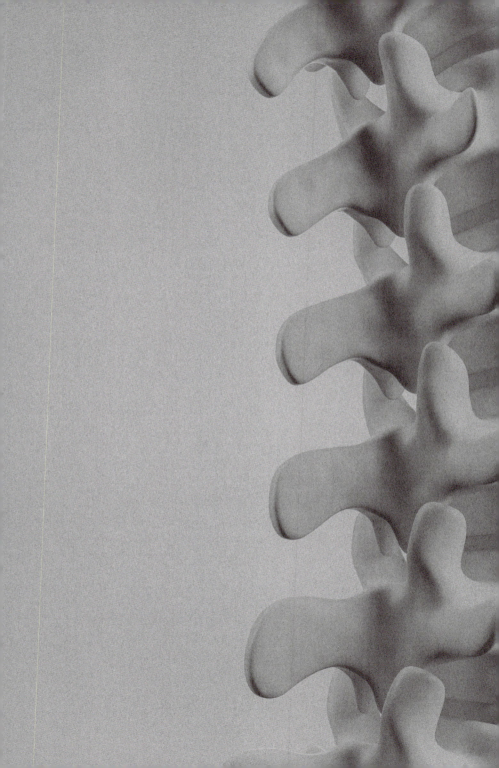

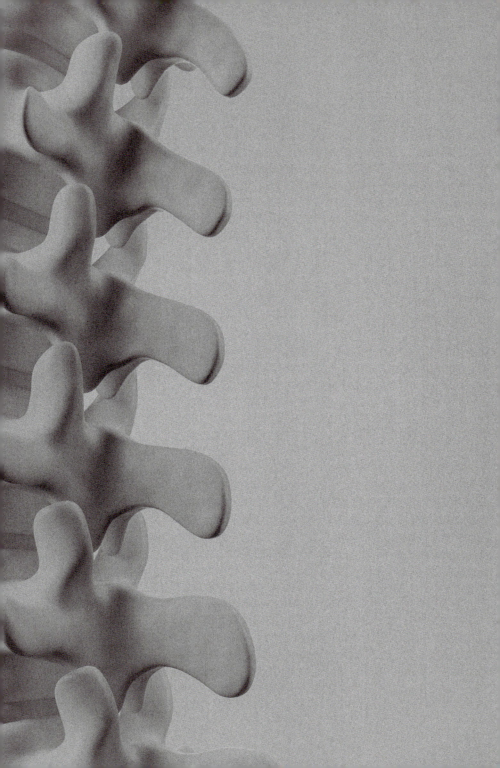

PART 2

A SURGICAL PERSPECTIVE ON THE THORACIC SPINE

1. SURGICAL APPROACHES TO THE THORACIC SPINE

The thoracic spine can be surgically approached from the anterior (ventral) or posterior (dorsal). In the posterior approach, a midline incision is made and the thoracolumbar fascia is opened at the midline, to then dissect between the muscles and the bone anatomy of the posterior spine. The spinous processes are exposed, as well as the laminae and one can dissect further laterally to expose the transverse processes and even further to the costotransverse junction and onto the ribs. Sometimes a transmuscular approach is performed by making an incision 5-6cm lateral to the midline in order to open the thoracolumbar fascia more laterally and arrive at the rib and transverse process. From there, a costotransversectomy can be performed.

The anterior approach to the thoracic spine is more elaborate. Such an approach can be achieved by opening the thorax laterally in between two ribs (thoracotomy) or introducing endoscopic ports in between ribs (thoracoscopy) and deflating one lung to arrive at the lateral side of the thoracic spine. This approach allows access from T5 to T12. The surgeon will choose the right or left route based on the anatomy of the surrounding structures (liver, aorta) and on the exact location of the target. The scapula precludes easy access above T5, unless one mobilises the scapula, which is associated with postoperative functional shoulder muscle morbidity. When access to the cranial thoracic spine is required and the patient's anatomy allows for it, a cervical approach just above the sternum may allow to reach to T2. If not, and to get to T3 and T4, a trans-sternal approach is required, with the help of a cardiac surgeon.

The posterior approach is definitely less invasive than a thoracotomy or trans-sternal approach, and the stiff thoracic spine also accommodates too much postoperative pain from muscle manipulation, but it prevents an accurate view to deal with extradural processes in front of the thecal sac. When this is required, an anterior approach should be chosen. The invasiveness of a thoracotomy is in the inevitable pneumothorax (for which a postoperative thorax tube is required) and postoperative costalgia (from pulling on the ribs or breaking them). This can be diminished by endoscopic surgery (thoracoscopy), but the gain is not indefinite. A trans-sternal approach is only very rarely needed and one should be careful to avoid serious vascular complications.

So, what can a surgeon achieve in the thoracic spine? Surgery can be indicated to reduce tumour or infection load. In addition, surgery can decompress the spinal cord, or – rarely required – an intercostal nerve because of radicular pain. The need for arthrodesis in the stiff thoracic spine will depend on the extent of bone resection required: if the decompression or debulking/resection introduces instability, the surgery will include stabilisation by osteosynthesis and – in many instances – bone fusion. Of note, this is not necessarily the case. Thoracic disc herniation surgery, for instance, will include only little bone resection and no arthrodesis. Also, thoracic laminectomy is less prone to kyphotic deformity in the stiffer thoracic spine than in the cervical spine, although it may occur. Besides decompressive objectives, the thoracic spine can be involved in thoracolumbar (kypho)scoliotic deformities that one wants to correct and stabilise. Also in trauma surgery, stabilisation without need for decompression may be aimed for. In the thoracic spine, the latter will not necessarily be associated with bone fusion, because after healing of the fracture, one may consider removing the hardware.

2. TRAUMA OF THE THORACIC SPINE

At the scene of the accident and when the situation is safe and the victim is resuscitated, the victim will preferably be immobilised to prevent any potential undue movement of parts of the spine that could endanger the spinal cord. This rule is valid for the entire spine. However, whereas most centres have rules for formal clearing of the cervical spine after any accident, further investigation and clearing of the thoracic spine will only be performed when there are clinical clues pointing at thoracic spinal injury, such as bruises at inspection, pain at palpation or tapping, or neurological deficits. CT-scanning will be the imaging modality of choice, while X-ray may be sufficient only in the situation of an older patient with suspected osteoporosis having developed pain after a brisk movement or minor trauma (the osteoporotic compression fractures resulting from low injury are stable injuries). Ligamentous injuries are less frequent in the thoracic spine, and it will actually be fierce displacement of bone parts on the CT scan that will point at it. Therefore, MRI will hardly be needed here (unless in bamboo spine patients to obtain full assessment of the subtle injury that is prone to extend over all 3 columns and then is unstable).

General principles on spine injury management are similar to the cervical spine. Lesions that are considered unstable should be surgically stabilised, whereas stable injuries can be immobilised in a brace. Stability will again be assessed by parameters such as type, location and extent of the fracture within the Dennis 3-column concept (anterior, middle and posterior column), vertebral body height loss, kyphotic angulation and fracture comminution. Cord compression by disrupted bone fragments or spine displacement (luxation) requires decompression or reduction, and subsequent stabilisation. Ligamentous injuries in the thoracic spine will usually be associated with disruption and displacement.

Thoracic spine injuries are classified according to the Magerl classification. Type A fractures result from vertebral body compression. They are referred to as 'burst fracture' when the anterior and middle column are involved. Stability of burst fractures depends on height loss, kyphotic angle and comminution, and also in case of bone protrusion compressing the spinal cord they will be operated on. Type B fractures are characterised by the disruption of the anterior or posterior tension band and are unstable injuries. Type C fractures involve displacement in any direction and are seriously unstable. Surgery will usually include posterior stabilisation by pedicle screws and intraoperative reduction (by distraction or 'ligamentotaxis'). When the body is not capable of providing sufficient anterior column support any longer, anterior body removal and reconstruction may be required, which will usually be performed in a second stage. The thoracolumbar junction area is the most frequent location of thoracolumbar injuries.

Also in thoracic spine trauma, the spinal cord can get injured. After emergency spinal cord decompression and stabilisation, patients with spinal cord injury belong on the intensive care ward in order to ensure sufficiently high blood pressure, as stated earlier. Depending on the level of spinal cord injury, thoracic spinal cord injury patients are less prone to respiratory problems than their cervical counterparts, and autonomous function may be largely spared in more caudal injuries when most of the cornu laterale and brain communication to it remains intact. Also, in terms of autonomy, for leisure and professional activity, having intact arm function means a great deal, as opposed to cervical spinal cord injury patients.

Be aware that, as stated previously, a patient with ankylosing spondylitis and spinal pain following even minor trauma has a fracture until otherwise proven. Osteoporotic fractures are usually type A injuries that only involve the anterior column and can be considered as stable, prone to heal spontaneously. In such a situation, Kahler's disease (multiple myeloma) should be ruled out by a protein electrophoresis, and all attention should go to comfort by adequate painkillers and physiotherapy to restore activity to the best level possible. When pain persists over six weeks or longer, vertebroplasty (injection of cement inside the collapsed vertebral body) may offer help. For the two latter situations, the context can mislead the caregiver, since the traumatic event is sometimes minor and not always identifiable.

3. THORACIC DISC HERNIATION

Thoracic disc herniations are one of the strangest and most intriguing phenomena in the spine. They may be soft as in cervical and lumbar disc herniations, which consist of herniated nucleus pulposus, but most often they are calcified. They can be really large, like pieces of bone that point into the spinal cord. Their origin is unknown, since the calcified herniations are totally different from the cervical and lumbar protrusions that result from an annular defect.

Thoracic disc herniations may cause severe spinal cord compression and subsequent myelopathic symptoms such as gait problems due to proprioception deficits (ataxia), weakness and/or spasticity and sphincter disturbances in terms of urinary urge or urge incontinence and constipation. Symptoms may evolve slowly, but in some instances they develop over days or weeks. Thoracic disc herniations that are located more laterally in the canal may provoke radicular pain over the rib. Whether or not they can be responsible for dorsalgia is a matter of debate. In most cases of dorsalgia, physiotherapy can relieve the complaint, proving the herniation is not related to the mechanical pain. Moreover, spinal cord compression does not result in any pain. In many instances, they are diagnosed as an incidental finding on an MRI scan that was ordered for a totally different reason, and hence, are asymptomatic.

Management depends on symptoms. Obvious and incapacitating myelopathic symptoms or progressive myelopathic symptoms represent a clear indication for surgery. Since the calcified disc herniations are usually very adherent to the thecal sac, any attempt to remove them from the posterior is inappropriate and even dangerous. Many reports exist of patients with severe neurological deficits including paraplegia after such endeavour. Non-calcified disc herniations may be removed through a costotransversectomy approach, but particularly in calcified herniations a thoracotomy (or thoracoscopic) approach is the preferred and safer option. A small box space is created by drilling the posterior part of the disc and a small portion of the upper and lower vertebrae in order to gently dissect and pull the calcified disc herniation away from the thecal sac into the drilled box. As this box is small, no arthrodesis is required.

One may be in equipoise as to whether or not a thoracic disc herniation causing radicular pain (over the rib) should be surgically treated, because thoracotomy or thoracoscopy is associated with a certain percentage of postoperative costalgia. In other words, the net result may be that one pain is replaced by the other. Fortunately, in my experience, radicular pain is rare, and often resolved by transforaminal injections by an experienced pain therapist. Axial pain is most likely not related to the diagnosed thoracic disc herniation, and literature advocates against surgery in those cases. Rehabilitation by well-trained physiotherapists that can deal with costovertebral joint problems and any other dorsalgia problem is the far better option here. When a large herniation compressing the spinal cord is found in a patient without symptoms and signs of myelopathy, one should explain symptoms that should alert the patient to swiftly see an expert neurosurgeon, and following up on the patient a couple of times for a clinical neuro examination may be wise.

4. YELLOW LIGAMENT HYPERTROPHY

More often in people with an Asian background than in Caucasians (or others), myelopathic symptoms and signs may be provoked by ossification and hypertrophy of the yellow ligament at one or more thoracic levels, hence compressing the thecal sac and spinal cord from the posterior. The calcified ligament usually is highly adherent to the thecal sac and tears may arise during decompressive surgery that is

performed through a posterior laminectomy approach. When carefully performed, the outcome is usually comparable to cervical degenerative myelopathy: surgery can arrest the progressive deterioration, but
many patients do improve neurologically.

5. OTHER THAN TRAUMATIC AND DEGENERATIVE CONDITIONS

The conditions described here are red flag conditions, most of them
being rather rare. The physiotherapist should be able to detect and
refer such conditions (see chapter 8) appropriately. However, the patient's trajectory does not stop there. Red flag situations may lead to
surgery and hence, may require postoperative physiotherapy.

Due to its large cumulative volume of intravertebral bone marrow,
the thoracic spine is the most frequent region where pathologies that
spread via a haematogenous route occur. Hence, spinal metastases
and spondylodiscitis are most often seen in the thoracic spine. As outlined in chapter 5 of the cervical spine, patients with spinal metastasis and unstable pathological fractures and/or (imminent) spinal cord
compression are candidates for surgical stabilisation or debulking
and stabilisation, followed by radiotherapy. Primary malignant bone
tumours can also occur in the thoracic spine, and the thoracic anatomy enables complete en bloc resection in selected cases by means of a
'spondylectomy', during which (part of) the lamina is removed and the
rest of the vertebra is released and flipped out taking care not to damage the spinal cord and not to breach the tumour's capsule. En bloc
surgery in some of these tumours (eg. sarcomas) drastically reduces
recurrence rate and improves chances of progression free survival.

Also for infections, I refer to chapter 5 in the cervical spine text. Whenever the infection has caused instability and/or symptomatic spinal
cord compression or when the patient is so severely ill that the infectious source should be removed surgically, patients are eligible for surgical stabilisation (arthrodesis) and/or decompression (corpectomy or
laminectomy). Following accurate debridement and under targeted

antibiotics, instrumentation hardware can be safely used, even in infection cases.

Deformity of the thoracic spine may be part of a scoliosis (adolescent idiopathic scoliosis in youngsters and degenerative scoliosis in adults), kyphosis (Scheuermann in youngsters, degenerative in adults), or a combination of both. Such conditions require specific expertise regarding evolution and operative possibilities. When a patient has chronic or progressive dysfunction and the inspection reveals a deformity, expert advice from an orthopaedic department with experience in spinal deformity surgery is recommended. In selective cases, deformity correction surgery may be warranted.

6. POSTOPERATIVE REHABILITATION

No studies report on the role and benefit of postoperative rehabilitation specifically in the context of thoracic spine surgery. As stated in the chapters on cervical spine surgery, in general, there should be no refrain from activation and at least a couple of postoperative physiotherapy contacts are useful to counsel and coach the patient and accommodate their worries, beliefs and practical questions. Although the thoracic spine is rather stiff, as opposed to the cervical and lumbar spine, patients can have muscular pain and anterior surgery may be associated with costovertebral issues. When it is safe to start physiotherapy following surgery, again, is an open question. In most instances, either there will be no stability issues or arthrodesis will have been applied when stability was an issue. This means that after a short period of soft tissue healing, starting exercises is very likely to be safe. The only situation in which it is reasonable to wait for bone healing is in compression fractures that are managed conservatively. Many of these patients will be braced, although we must admit that there is no evidence whatsoever on the usefulness and effectiveness of bracing. In this period of bone healing, conditioning exercises of stabilisers and posture may be considered. When it is considered that the bracing can stop, it may be useful to gradually taper down the duration of bracing during the day, in order to allow the muscles to gradually regain condition.

7. WHAT ABOUT AXIAL PAIN?

Axial pain is not an indication for surgery. As opposed to the cervical and lumbar spine where a tendency exists in more aggressive surgeons to swiftly offer arthrodesis surgery in axial pain, in spite of evidence and guidelines, this is less the case for thoracic axial pain. Some surgeons are overly aggressive in surgically treating thoracic disc herniations associated with axial pain and without myelopathy. As stated earlier, the overall triage concept outlined in the introduction of this book offers a practical guideline. Red flags should be ruled out first, and dorsalgia is considered somewhat a red flag on its own. The reason for this is that the thoracic spine is less prone to degeneration than the cervical and lumbar spine (but may still run into overload problems, of course), and that haematogenous spread of tumours or infections finds a predilection site in the thoracic spine. Importantly, red flags should be interpreted in clusters, and not every patient with dorsalgia has a serious underlying disease. In that regard, it is helpful to investigate whether or not the dorsalgia has mechanical characteristics, i.e. better in rest and worse during or following physical loading. Radicular pain is very rare in the thoracic spine.

As for non-red flag mechanical axial pain, the management depends on the timeline: the further a patient proceeds in time, the more should be invested in addressing psychosocial risk factors and in avoiding chronicity. In chronic thoracic pain, rehabilitation potential and all relevant risk factors should be carefully assessed, and in my opinion specialists in physical medicine are in the best position to do this. In case of deformity and persistent problems, it may be useful to ask for an expert orthopaedic surgery consult.

8. RED FLAGS IN THE THORACIC SPINE

RUPTURED AORTA ANEURYSM	• Man > 50 years with vascular risk factors: smoking, arterial hypertension, hyper-cholesterolemia, diabetes mellitus … • Intense pain in the back as well as in the abdomen, often radiation in the L3 dermatome is reported • Unwell, shock • Pulsating abdominal mass
MYELOPATHY	• Gait instability, atactic or spastic gait • Weakness in the lower limbs • Hypoesthesia in the trunk and/or lower limbs • Urinary urge or urge incontinence, neurogenic bladder, constipation • Hyperreflexia in the lower limbs, pathological cutaneous reflexes and Babinski signs, hypertonia and spastic paraparesis
INFECTIOUS DISORDER	• Severe and continuous dorsalgia • Pain worse at night, pain that is not affected by position or movement • Fever, chills • Recent gastro-intestinal/gynaecological infection or surgery • Recent thoracic spine surgery • Immune suppression • Intravenous drug use • Recent bacterial infection • Older age

INFLAMMATORY PAIN	• Morning stiffness • Pain at rest, less pain during movement • Pain at night, particularly in the second half of the night • Pain when tired
OSTEOPOROTIC COMPRESSION FRACTURE	• Sudden onset axial pain after a brisk movement or (even minor) trauma in patient known or suspected with osteoporosis or long-term steroid use • New onset structural spinal deformity • Severe pain, pain better when lying down
TRAUMATIC FRACTURE	• Sudden onset of pain and possibility of traumatic event • New onset structural spinal deformity • Severe pain, pain better when lying down • Known or suspected ankylosing spondylitis or DISH and onset of dorsalgia following (even minor) trauma (= fracture until otherwise proven)
SPINAL TUMOUR	• New onset dorsalgia in a patient older than 50 years (55 years in some guidelines) or younger than 20 years • History of cancer • Persistent pain, pain worse at night, pain that is not affected by position or movement • New onset structural spinal deformity • Pain in different locations • Unexplained weight loss

PANCREATITIS	• Pain in the upper abdomen radiating to the back • Alcohol abuse, cholecystolithiasis, hypercalcaemia • Following ERCP procedure or abdominal trauma
GALL STONE CRISIS (GALL COLIC)	• Episodic pains in the upper right abdomen, often following meals • Pain may radiate to the midback or shoulders • Urge to move, nausea, vomiting • Icterus (yellow skin), light-coloured stools
PULMONARY PATHOLOGY (PNEUMONIA, PLEURAL EFFUSION, EMPYEMA, PNEUMOTHORAX)	• Pain when breathing, thoracic pain and/or dorsalgia • Dyspnea • Cough, illness, feeling unwell, fever
CARDIAC PATHOLOGY (ISCHAEMIA, PERICARDITIS)	• Heavy, unsettling, tight feeling in the thorax, possibly radiating to the shoulders, arms, midback • Unwell, paleness, nausea, transpiration, dyspnea • Sudden onset pain, not responding to painkillers

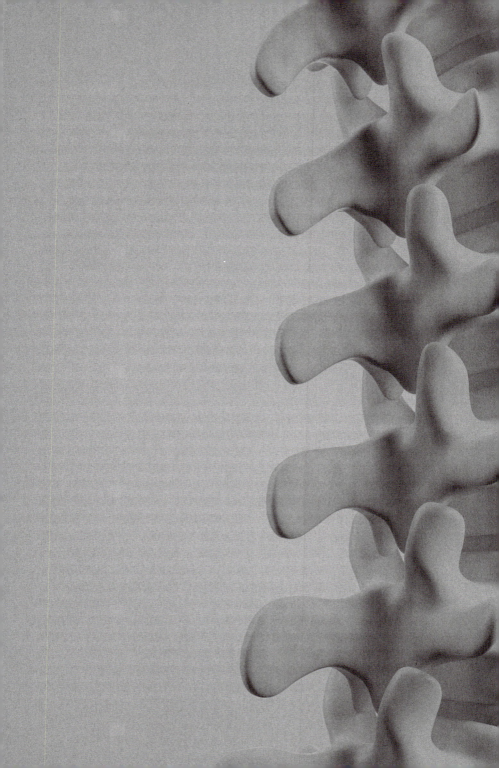

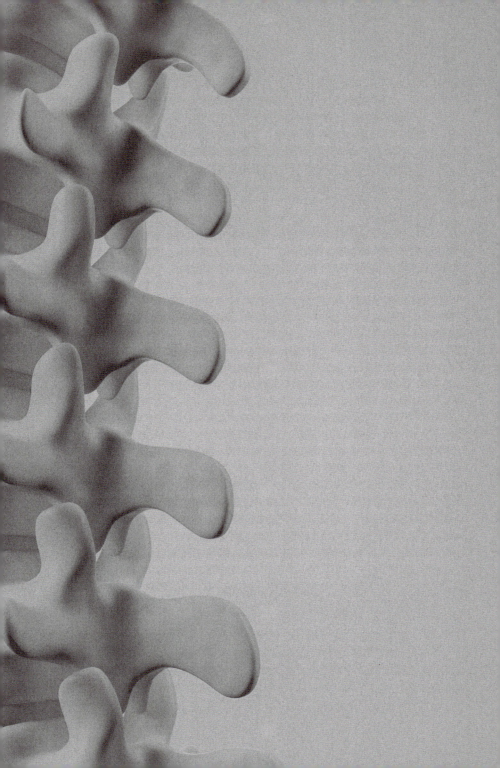

PART 3

A SURGICAL PERSPECTIVE ON THE LUMBOSACRAL SPINE

1. SURGICAL APPROACHES TO THE LUMBOSACRAL SPINE

In general, the lumbosacral spine can be approached from posterior or anterior, actually meaning posterior to the plane of transverse processes and intertransverse ligaments, or anterior to it. The 'classic' posterior approach is the midline approach in which the thoracolumbar fascia is divided at or just lateral from the supraspinous ligaments, to further dissect the muscles away from the spinous processes, laminae and facet joints (or even further laterally). Interestingly, the multifidus muscles are attached to the laminae and on the motion level of the facet joints and discs, there is a fatty plane that allows separation of the muscles from the midline without interrupting their midline attachment. This is in fact also true in the cervical and thoracic spine, but in the lumbar spine this fatty plane has a larger volume, useful in single level approaches. As a whole, the layers of lumbar spine muscles represent a huge and strong mass of muscle tissue that is hard to push aside. Very often, neuromuscular blocking agents are being used during this dissection allowing muscle retraction, and long-lasting retraction may cause damage by provoking muscle ischaemia. As an alternative to the classic midline approach, paramedian transmuscular routes have been developed, in which muscle fibres are split, or a plane between muscle bundles is followed, leaving midline attachments intact (the so-called Wiltse approach). There is certainly a theoretical benefit to the latter, but a positive effect on long-term function surprisingly has never been proven.

The anterior route has many faces, is always extraperitoneal, and in principle consists of 1) a true anterior view at L4 to S1 (through a Pfannenstiel or infra-umbilical vertical incision and dissecting along the peritoneum on one side over the psoas muscle to push the peritoneal sac to the contralateral side and enabling straight working channels beneath the iliac vessel bifurcation at L5S1 or lateral to the large vessels at L4L5) or 2) a straight lateral to anterolateral oblique view at L1 to L4 (through a lateral to more anterolateral incision, minimally invasive or open, and retroperitoneal dissection onto the spine). The latter always includes a dissection of the psoas muscle, pushing it posteriorly or anteriorly depending on what angle one is coming from and taking care not to harm the lumbosacral plexus that runs in an oblique fashion from cranial-posterior to caudal-anterior.

The posterior approaches provide a good view on the thecal sac and nerve roots (and the thecal sac containing cauda equina can be mobilised without risk for neurological injury as opposed to the spinal cord higher up), but is associated with more muscle manipulation and associated pain and dysfunction. The anterior routes provide a better view onto the vertebral bodies and discs, but are associated with a risk for vessel injury, autonomous plexus injury and lumbosacral plexus injury.

So, what can a surgeon achieve in the lumbosacral spine? Surgery can be indicated to reduce tumour or infection load. In addition, surgery can decompress the conus of the spinal cord (in the upper lumbar spine) or cauda equina (lower down) or one or more nerve roots in the lateral recess, foramen or extraforaminal space. When a facet joint needs to be removed to accomplish the decompression of a nerve root, arthrodesis will be required (consisting of osteosynthesis and bone fusion). Laminectomy in the lumbar spine will interrupt the posterior tension band and may accelerate degenerative changes and deformities in the long run, and therefore as a singular technique it is largely abandoned and replaced by interlaminar decompression techniques preserving laminae and the midline.

On the other hand, arthrodesis for exclusion of motion can be achieved. This may be required in trauma situations (preferably osteosynthesis or internal fixation without bone fusion because after healing of the fracture removal of the hardware can restore mobility). In addition, arthrodesis is sometimes aimed for in the belief that it will prevent abnormal motion in degenerated joints and thereby provide pain relief. In the latter situation, surgeons will aim for osteosynthesis and bone fusion. What about restoring motion? Disc prostheses were intended to restore motion and improve back pain in disc degeneration, but this new motion is non-physiological and until now the long-term benefit over conservative treatment for degenerative disc disease has not been proven. Therefore, they are largely abandoned. Finally, the lumbar spine can be involved in thoracolumbar (kypho)scoliotic deformities that one wants to correct and stabilise in deformity surgery.

2. TRAUMA OF THE LUMBOSACRAL SPINE

For initial management, diagnosis, general principles and classification, trauma of the lumbar spine is similar to the thoracic spine (see chapter 2, thoracic spine): immobilisation for transport, CT scan imaging upon clinical suspicion (X-ray may be sufficient when an osteoporotic fracture is suspected), most injuries being bone fractures and ligamentous injury being rare (an example is the ligamentous anteroposterior injury typically above or below L3 and associated with abdominal injury seen in high velocity car accidents and called 'seat belt injury'), surgical stabilisation for 'unstable injuries' and immobilisation for 'stable injuries' including the way we assess 'stability', bone fragments compressing the conus or cauda equina needing to be removed followed by surgical stabilisation, and finally, the use of the same Magerl classification. As stated earlier, the thoracolumbar junction area is the most frequent site of traumatic injuries in the thoracolumbar spine. Sacral fractures usually occur as part of pelvic fractures, which is not the subject of this book.

Compression of the thecal sac in the lumbar spine will not lead to the 'typical' spinal cord injury (upper motor injury below the lesion), but to conus injuries in the upper lumbar spine and cauda equina injuries in the lower lumbar and sacral spine. This may result in urinary retention, constipation, saddle anaesthesia and sexual dysfunction with – depending on the level – combinations of lower limb muscle weakness (lower motor neuron injury) and regions of hypo/anaesthesia.

As stated previously, a patient with ankylosing spondylitis and lumbar pain following even minor trauma has a fracture until otherwise proven. Osteoporotic fractures can occur in the entire lumbar spine and are usually stable type A injuries that are prone to spontaneous healing. Emphasis is on offering comfort and preserving activity after ruling out multiple myeloma. If pain persists over several weeks, vertebroplasty can be considered. On the same note, patients with osteoporosis can suffer from sacral insufficiency fractures that can be extremely painful but usually heal with conservative therapy. It is something that should be in the differential diagnosis when an older person (particularly female) develops severe pain in the lower back to pelvis. In all situations of the current paragraph, the traumatic event may be so minor that people even have forgotten it.

3. LUMBAR DISC HERNIATION

The etiology of lumbar radicular pain is similar to that in the cervical spine and was outlined in chapter 3. Disc herniations are a prominent cause of lumbar radicular pain. They result from weakened spots in the posterior annulus fibrosus which in turn result from numerous episodes of increased intradiscal pressure in the posterior half of the disc during lumbar flexion movements (bending over) and positions (sitting). From weakened annular areas, defects arise, through where the nucleus pulposus can extrude into the canal. In most instances, the posterior longitudinal ligament will prevent the herniated nucleus part from moving freely inside the spinal canal, but will not prevent it from exerting static compression and dynamic irritation of the nerve root that lies there. It is believed that dural irritation can provoke back pain, while it is known for certain that nerve root irritation does result in radicular pain. I often tell my patients that the annular layers are similar to onion layers: when you cut a hole, the edges cannot be pulled together. In other words, once there is an annular defect, this will not heal spontaneously nor can it be closed surgically.

There are numerous terminologies to classify disc herniations in terms of their size and containment by the posterior ligament. In fact, this is not really relevant from a clinical perspective. What does matter is the exact location of the disc herniation. While in the cervical spine, the anatomy is small and a disc herniation with or without associated osteophytes in a paramedian or lateral position will inevitably irritate the same exiting nerve root of that motion level, the lumbar anatomy is different because of its larger vertebrae. As a result, the exiting nerve root of a particular motion level (wearing the number of the upper vertebra) will only cross the disc of that particular level in the lateral half of the foramen and extraforaminal zone. At the same time, the nerve root that will exit at the level below (wearing the number of the lower vertebra) will also cross that same disc, more in particular where that nerve root branches off the thecal sac (i.e. its shoulder). As a consequence, disc herniations in a paramedian position (most frequent) will compress and irritate the nerve root that exits on the level below, whereas more lateral disc herniations (intra- to extraforaminal;

less often) will compress and irritate the nerve root of the level itself. When interventional therapy for incapacitating or persistent radicular pain is considered, this is very important, since the imaging should match the clinical picture of the radicular pattern. If not consistent, no intervention should be undertaken and diagnostic work to reveal the true cause of symptoms should be continued.

A lumbar disc herniation causing nerve root irritation will lead to radicular pain in the leg: lancinating, shooting, sometimes incredible pain. It may arise suddenly, sometimes after a 'wrong' movement such as a brisk torsion movement, but can also install itself gradually. As stated earlier, radicular pain has 3 characteristics. It is associated with a pattern in many cases, and that pattern more or less coincides with the dermatome of the involved root. Most disc herniations occur at L4L5 and L5S1 (the lowest levels in the lumbar spine), resulting in L5 and S1 being the most frequently affected nerve roots. Next, radicular pain can be provoked. For lumbar radicular pain of discogenic origin, provocation is by lumbar flexion (bending over, sitting), nerve root stretching (straight leg raise test, Bragard's sign), increasing intraspinal pressure (Valsalva manoeuvres such as coughing and sneezing, which increases venous pressure also in the epidural venous plexus) and compression (quadratus lumborum, gluteal muscles). Be aware that none of these tests bears absolute sensitivity nor specificity. Finally, there may be associated neurological symptoms ('radiculopathy'): tingling and/or hypoesthesia in the dermatome, muscle weakness and/or hypo- to areflexia in the involved myotome. Back pain may be associated, but this is variable and non-specific.

Large disc herniations that also compress the S2 to S4 rootlets may cause saddle numbness, urinary retention, constipation and sexual dysfunction, along with the associated uni- or bilateral radicular pain and potential weakness and numbness. This is named the cauda equina syndrome (because all roots of the cauda equina are compressed); representing a medical emergency (and is therefore an absolute red flag): if decompression is not performed within hours, sphincter and sexual dysfunction remain. A typical story begins with enormous back pain, followed somewhat later by radicular pain. Shortly after, the devastating neurological symptoms arise, and at that point, the back pain and radicular pain often decrease. The patient therefore thinks he is already getting better and is not too alarmed. Nevertheless, urinary retention (by parasympathetic dysfunction) and saddle numbness are the hallmarks that should be picked up accurately by every caregiver.

Differential diagnosis includes other radicular problems, plexus conditions, joint conditions, tendon conditions, vascular conditions and peripheral nerve conditions. An intradural tumour on the conus or more caudally on the cauda equina may provoke very similar symptoms to a disc herniation, albeit it that the straight leg raise test may not be positive and that the pain may be worse at night. Stenotic radicular compression will be dealt with in a next chapter. Also extradural spinal tumours and epidural abscesses may manifest themselves with a radicular pain component, besides more or less pronounced red flag symptoms (weight loss, fever, pain at night, being unwell ...). At each patient contact red flags should be screened again. Inflammatory radicular conditions include Lyme's disease and herpes zoster (zona). Lumbosacral plexus inflammation can result from peridiverticulitis, although this is a very rare condition. Plexus compression may arise from pelvic tumours, such as ovary tumours, but also neurogenic tumours such as Schwannomas or neurofibromas. In plexus conditions neuropathic pain and neurological symptoms may be more dominant than in discogenic shooting radicular pain.

Next, sacroiliac, hip- and knee-related pain and dysfunction can be investigated by their typical history of load- and movement-associated pain and the clinical provocation tests. Chronic gluteal tendinitis problems, usually in elderly patients, present in the hip and thigh region and are associated with painful palpation. Arterial insufficiency is associated with effort-induced gluteal or calf pain, so-called vascular claudication, and should be differentiated from neurogenic claudication resulting from lumbar spinal canal stenosis, which is explained in the next chapter.

Peroneal neuropathy resulting from compression and irritation of the common peroneal nerve at the fibular head leads to foot drop and eversion weakness. Inversion weakness allows one to differentiate: when it is present, it points at an L5 radicular origin of the foot drop. Peroneal neuropathy results from external compression (plaster immobilisation, long knee-crossed sitting, long squatting) or substantial weight loss. Whereas in L5 compression the foot drop is usually associated with radicular pain at onset, pain is not a major symptom in peroneal neuropathy. This is different in peripheral nerve tumours (Schwannomas, neurofibromas) that can be painful, but there again, tingling and other associated neurological symptoms will usually be dominant.

Polyneuropathy, eg. in diabetes or following chemotherapy, results in tingling and numbness in (glove and) sock distribution, potentially with neuropathic (i.e. burning, warm, cold) pain. Finally, some referred pains from lumbar muscular or articular origin are referred to as pseudoradicular pain. To diagnose the latter, other conditions should be ruled out. Pseudoradicular leg pain always stays above the knee.

General management of lumbar radicular pain according to the timeline is extensively explained in the chapter on cervical radicular pain. In short, in acute (less than 6 weeks) radicular pain one will check strength and cauda equina symptoms (swiftly refer in case of deficit) and psychosocial risk factors (as from 2 weeks). Management will be conservative (unless weakness or cauda equina syndrome), with accurate explanation of the high chances of spontaneous improvement and reassurance, comfort measures and promotion of staying active. There is no need for imaging when weakness, cauda equina syndrome and red flags are ruled out. Patients with risk factors will be followed up more closely and offered education and coaching, for which the physiotherapist is well placed. Graded exercises may be useful to help the patient back to the premorbid status. Again, while often helpful, the role of more specific physiotherapy actions is still unclear. When pain is too cumbersome and while awaiting spontaneous resolution, fluoroscopically guided steroid injection is an option.

In the subacute stage (6-12 weeks), in addition to the above, surgery can be offered as an option, and knowledge about this option is one of the points of this book. Neuropathic pain characteristics may warrant prescription of anti-neuropathic drugs. In the chronic stage (12 weeks and longer) a surgery consult is strongly advisable. This does not mean that the patient should necessarily be operated on, but the patient is entitled to a surgical expert opinion. Usually, I show patients the graphs from the 2007 randomised controlled Leiden-The Hague disc herniation trial: at 6-8 weeks after onset surgery leads to fast relief of pain, but at 1 year leg pain scores are similar in operated and non-operated patients. In a more recent randomised trial in patients with 4-6 months of radicular pain, pain scores another 6 months later were significantly lower in the surgery group.

The goal of disc herniation surgery is to relieve the radicular symptoms. In over 90 percent of patients that were correctly diagnosed, radicular pain scores drop significantly immediately or shortly after surgery. In addition, recovery of muscle weakness may be swift when surgical decompression is done within hours (to a couple of days maximum) of appearance. Recovery of numbness is usually very slow (with or without surgery: sensory deficit on its own is not an indication for surgery). Recovery of back pain is variable and unpredictable, and back pain on its own is considered a poor indication for surgery.

Lumbar disc herniation surgery is simpler than cervical surgery. There is no spinal cord to take into account when deciding on the preferred route, and the thecal sac containing cauda equina can be retracted without risk. All lumbar disc herniation surgery is performed from the back, either through a midline approach and opening up the fatty paramedian plane at the interlaminar level, or through a Wiltse approach, slightly more lateral and going transmuscular. Loupe magnification or microscope magnification is used. Next, the yellow ligament is opened and resected, the thecal sac and nerve root are identified, mobilised and gently retracted medially over the herniation. The posterior longitudinal ligament is then opened and the herniated nucleus pulposus removed.

In the past, this was completed with a 'discectomy', meaning that the surgeon would pass through the annular defect with biopsy forceps to empty as much of the nucleus pulposus (note that in this type of surgery 'discectomy' has a slightly different meaning than in anterior surgery where it means that the entire disc including annulus is removed). Nowadays, since it has been demonstrated that discectomy does not reduce the incidence of recurrence as compared with sequestrectomy, usually only sequestrectomy is performed, i.e. only the herniated part is removed, leaving the disc itself untouched. As explained, the annular defect is like a hole cut in an onion: the edges cannot be brought together. Several devices have been tried out to enable closing the defect during surgery, however without success. As a consequence, risk of recurrence is inevitably associated with disc herniation surgery, incidences in literature being on average 10 percent over the course of several years.

Complications of lumbar discectomy or sequestrectomy are infrequent. Nerve root injury or postoperative hematoma with potential weakness, and abdominal vessel injury by damaging the anterior annulus all have incidences of far less than 1 percent. The risk for postoperative infection (discitis) lies around 2 percent (and should be carefully managed with biopsy or debridement and accurately targeted antibiotics). The risk for a dural tear is on average 5 percent, is usually appropriately dealt with during the surgery itself and rarely leads to additional surgery or associated complications (headache, pseudomeningocele, fistula and meningitis). In all series, a certain subset of patients – usually 5-10% – has less favourable results in terms of radicular pain relief or develops additional back pain. These patients usually also score higher on psychosocial risk factors.

Patients can be immediately mobilised. In North America, disc surgery is often performed in a day surgery setting. When we initiated such a programme in Leuven, we were happy to learn that this was perfectly possible and meant no disadvantage for long-term results. In most centres, patients will be discharged the day after surgery. There is some evidence on postoperative rehabilitation, mostly showing that early rehabilitation – as from two weeks – is safe and a couple of studies were able to prove that early postoperative therapy was also associated with superior functional outcomes in the long run. As stated in the cervical radicular pain chapter, a postoperative physiotherapy consult on the ward is an absolute minimum. Most patients should be able to return to work within a couple of weeks, although the nature of the work should be taken into account. In case of hard physical labour, dedicated physiotherapy including work hardening is advocated. However, in my opinion, prescribing at least a couple of physiotherapy sessions (and more depending on findings), is helpful in all cases in order to guide coping and soft tissue healing, manage dysfunction and misbalance and optimise fitness for participation by training.

4. LUMBAR STENOSIS WITHOUT DEFORMITY

Similar to the cervical spine, natural degeneration processes in the lumbar spine will be associated with reduced disc height and disc bulging, but particularly with facet and yellow ligament hypertrophy. Three types (locations) of stenosis can be discerned and should be investigated on the imaging in patients with susceptible symptoms. In central stenosis, the thecal sac is being compressed from all sides by thickened yellow ligament, bigger facets, disc bulging and the posterior epidural fat layer. Typically, on a T2 axial MRI image, the nerve roots cannot be discriminated from one another with cerebrospinal fluid in between them any longer. In lateral recess stenosis, the sides of the canal in which the nerve roots branch off before entering the foramen are narrowed by yellow ligament and facet thickening, sometimes aggravated by disc bulging. This may occur without central stenosis, and should therefore be looked at separately, best to be identified on axial and sagittal T2 MRI images. Finally, the foramen can be narrowed. This may result from yellow ligament hypertrophy, that will then reduce the anteroposterior diameter at the entrance of the foramen. Alternatively, it may be the exit (lateral half) of the foramen that is narrowed in an anteroposterior direction by osteophytic spurs originating from the superior articular process (of the lower vertebra). And of course, combinations of medial and lateral foraminal stenosis may exist. Also, the foramen can be reduced in size secondary to deformities. Here, the nerve root will usually be compressed in a craniocaudal direction, which is discussed separately in chapter 6.

Lumbar spinal stenosis results in radicular pain, although the presentation is different from discogenic radicular pain. In principle, as in all radicular pains, the pain has a pattern and this may be very clear in monoradicular compression (eg. one foramen). However, many situations exist in which several roots are compressed at the same time (central stenosis, bilateral and multisegmental lateral recess stenosis), which will make the pattern less clear. Also, pain will often be described by the patient as sore, fatigue or cramping instead of shooting pain. Second, the pain can be provoked, but provocation is different from discogenic pain. The size of the canal and foramen are slightly smaller in extension and slightly larger in flexion. As a result, pain is provoked in lumbar extension, i.e. standing and walking. Patients will typically say that they can only walk a couple of hundred metres and then have to sit down, after which they can start over again. Resting in a standing position usually does not relieve the leg pain, since standing for a while will also provoke pain. This phenomenon is referred to as 'neurogenic claudication'. The good thing is that these patients are usually not in agony from their pain, because all they have to do for relief is sit down. Instead, their complaint will be that their mobility perimeter has drastically decreased, and interferes with their functional capabilities. At the same time, they can ride their bikes (if they still do) for tens of kilometres, and when they lean on the cart in the supermarket, they are as happy as can be. Finally, neurological symptoms can be associated, but since the compression installs only very gradually (as opposed to disc hernias), neurological symptoms and signs are actually very rare. Weakness resulting from stenosis is hardly ever seen.

I will not go into the differential diagnosis, which is explained in the previous chapter. Obviously, patients with stenosis are generally in their sixties and older, as opposed to the average age in disc herniation lying in the forties. Therefore, problems usually more often seen in the elderly are more prominent in the differential diagnosis, such as coxarthrosis, gluteal tendonitis and vascular claudication. Sometimes patients even have a combination of several etiologies contributing to their pain at the same time, and the challenge then is to identify what contributes more to the disability. Arterial insufficiency similarly leads to leg pain after walking a certain distance, but as opposed to neurogenic claudication this is swiftly relieved by standing still and the patient does not have to sit down. Inversely, patients with neurogenic claudication can perform in a bended position (walking with walking aid, pedal cycling), whereas vascular claudication patients cannot make such efforts without pain.

Management of neurogenic claudication perfectly fits within the timeline scheme outlined for radicular pain (see cervical radicular pain and lumbar disc hernation; also see www.lowbackpain.kce.be). However, what is characteristic of this condition is that it usually has a very gradual onset, and as patients get relief by sitting, they tend to only present at a chronic stage, i.e. with complaints existing for more than 3 months. In that stage, it would be unusual that the neurogenic claudication spontaneously resolves and surgical advice is advocated anyhow. It has been demonstrated in two trials (the Maine and the Sports trial) that surgery is superior to conservative management when the patient's mobility and quality of life is significantly impaired by the neurogenic claudication. As these patients are not in agony from debilitating pain and since steroid injections only offer temporary relief, they have only limited therapeutic value here, although they may be helpful for diagnostic reasons in some difficult pains that seem to have multiple origins. Hence, after confirming diagnosis and particularly ruling out vascular claudication and unless patients are only mildly affected or have significant comorbidities precluding surgery – in which case conservative management with physiotherapy counselling on accommodating activities and/or epidural injections is preferred – therapy will most often consist of surgical decompression. Still, as this concerns patient comfort and is not life-threatening, decisions are always being made in a shared decision making.

In the previous century, laminectomy was introduced by Verbiest as surgical treatment for this syndrome (spinal stenosis also being called 'Verbiest's syndrome'). This has been abandoned, since it is not the lamina that compresses the thecal sac, but the yellow ligaments and hypertrophic facet joints at motion level. Therefore, nowadays, standard surgery in lumbar stenosis consists of interlaminar decompression, i.e. the removal of yellow ligament in between two laminae, keeping the laminae, facet joints and midline (spinous processes and inter/supraspinous ligaments) intact. The latter helps to prevent long-term deformity from facet joint overloading that may occur after laminectomy (because the posterior tension band is removed). In the French language this type of surgery is called 'récalibrage', while the English often use the term 'laminotomy' to describe this operative technique. Interestingly, it is perfectly possible to bilaterally remove yellow ligament and hypertrophic bone to decompress the entire thecal sac and both lateral recesses by a unilateral approach.

The interlaminar decompression is the technique of choice for non-deformity stenosis and is able to decompress central stenosis, lateral recess stenosis and medial foraminal stenosis (foramen entry). For lateral foraminal stenosis (exit of the foramen), a transmuscular approach can be used to arrive at the lateral aspect of the facet joint and isthmus and remove the osteophyte arising from the superior articular process. Only in severe foraminal stenosis over the entire range of the foramen, it may be preferable to remove the facet joint, in which case arthrodesis will be required (see next chapter). It has been observed by many that some patients, in addition to reduction of neurogenic claudication by interlaminar decompression, also report reduction of back pain. However, performing decompressive surgery with the single purpose of relieving back pain, even in proven stenosis, is a too far stretch, as back pain usually has a multifactorial origin and no guarantee can be offered. Interlaminar decompression for stenosis in patients with neurogenic claudication is a gratifying activity: the large majority of patients report immediate or very fast resolution of symptoms, restoring their mobility perimeter.

Risk for complications is low. One should rule out alignment problems before surgery by performing a standing X-ray of the spine. Scans are always taken in a supine position and underestimate alignment problems (deformities), that may lead to different decisions, as will be explained in chapter 6. When this is forgotten and an unstable anterolisthesis or a scoliosis has been missed, decompression surgery might potentially lead to progressive deformity aggravation. Nerve root injury or bleeding complications leading to neurological deficits are rare (less than 1 percent). The most frequent complication, with an incidence of 5-10 percent on average, is a dural tear. Particularly older female patients can have very thin and fragile dura, increasing chances of an intraoperative tear, but this can usually be adequately repaired during the same surgery. When the problem persists, this may lead to intracranial hypotension headaches, a subcutaneous or subfascia pseudomeningocele or a cerebrospinal fluid fistula at worst. In most cases, this can be repaired in an additional surgery. As patients are usually a bit older and sometimes frail, postoperative infections or other medical complications may occur (such as pneumonia). Still, as the surgery is short and associated with very little blood loss, patients actually can be safely operated on up to a high age (including patients over 90 years of age).

Patients can be immediately mobilised following surgery. In the Leuven day surgery programme, not only lumbar disc herniation patients were included, but also lumbar stenosis patients. This worked perfectly fine, even in older patients. No proof of benefit of early physiotherapy exists, but it has been demonstrated to be safe (as from 2 weeks). Physiotherapy is helpful to accommodate kinesophobia or other false beliefs, counsel the patient on practical ADL issues, manage misbalance and dysfunction and make an early start with reconditioning.

5. LUMBAR SPINE ARTHRODESIS TECHNIQUES

At this point, and before engaging in deformities, let us explain how arthrodesis in the lumbar spine is achieved. Before the nineties of the previous century, arthrodesis was usually obtained by putting bone grafts in the gutter formed by the transverse processes and facet joints, and having the patient immobilised by a brace, since expertise and availability of hardware for osteosynthesis of the spine was not as widespread as it is now. The rate of insufficient healing of the bone (non-union) was relatively high. This improved when pedicle screws were introduced on a large scale, enabling direct and immediate immobility of the arthrodesis segment, and fusion rates got better. Still, often bone grafts eventually got absorbed by the surrounding muscles.

This was not necessarily problematic for the patient, because the osteo-synthesis hardware provided stability, but surgeons still were aiming at techniques that would also allow for higher effective fusion rates, as well as for possibilities to enable direct support in the anterior column closer to the axis of rotation.

This is where, after experimentation with intradiscal pieces of bone, the interbody cages were introduced: prefabricated struts in different sizes in PEEK or carbon that could be filled with bone grafts and insert-ed in the disc space after discectomy, and in which care has to be tak-en to sufficiently remove the endplate cartilage. A next step then was that in addition to the posterior technique of introducing cages, pro-cedures and cages were developed to be introduced from differently angled approaches. The character 'I' in the abbreviations that describe the fusion technique refers to 'interbody', i.e. discectomy and use of a cage for achievement of interbody fusion.

While the 'interbody' techniques are widely adopted and most popu-lar, in my view the posterior lumbar fusion (PLF) still has a great value when no anterior support or restoration of disc height is required. In 1948 McBride, an American surgeon, described that drilling out the facet joint gap and filling this gap with bone grafts provided an excel-lent means for effective fusion. Indeed, this has now been shown to be very effective when combined with screws, associated with high fusion rates. In a Scandinavian randomised trial posterior lumbar in-terbody fusion (PLIF) was not superior to PLF and PLF had fewer neu-rological complications.

In the PLIF procedure, two cages with bone or bone substitute are placed in the intervertebral space following discectomy (nucleus pul-posus and endplate cartilage) through a posterior interlaminar ap-proach, for each cage (right and left) by removing the inferior articular process of the upper level and retracting the thecal sac medially. This was soon followed by a modification of the technique, described as transforaminal lumbar interbody fusion (TLIF). Here, a cage with bone or bone substitute is placed in the intervertebral space following dis-cectomy (nucleus pulposus and endplate cartilage) through the foraminal area of the disc, i.e. in between the exiting nerve root of that level and the shoulder of the lower nerve root, which requires the resection of the entire facet joint at one side. The cage is then inserted in such a way that it crosses the midline, or multiple cages are inserted. The advantage of TLIF over PLIF is that less retraction on the thecal sac is required for cage insertion, and that the contralateral facet joint – that is not sacrificed – can be used for fusion as well. Minimally invasive techniques have been described that allow for facetectomy and TLIF through a transmuscular small cylindrical spreader.

On top of the posterior interbody techniques, procedures for cage introduction through routes anterior of the transverse process plane have been described. In ALIF (anterior lumbar interbody fusion) a cage with bone or bone substitute is placed in the intervertebral space following discectomy through an anterior abdominal (retroperitoneal) approach. This is possible at L4L5 and L5S1, and the iliac arteries and veins have to be carefully dissected and protected. In DLIF/XLIF (direct or extreme lateral interbody fusion) a cage is placed in the lumbar intervertebral space following discectomy through a lateral retroperitoneal trans-psoas approach, in which damage to the lumbosacral plexus needs to be carefully avoided. This is done at L1L2 to L4L5. To stay more anterior to the lumbosacral plexus, OLIF (oblique lumbar interbody fusion) was developed, in which a cage is placed in the intervertebral space following discectomy through an oblique anterior abdominal (retroperitoneal) approach, applicable at L1L2 to L4L5. Since the anterior techniques do not have to work around the thecal sac and exiting nerve roots, they allow for placing larger cages and thereby again increasing fusion rate. They also avoid posterior muscle manipulation. However, they need to take care of different important anatomical structures: the lumbosacral plexus, ureter, solar plexus and large arteries and veins.

Apart from potential complications originating from the different surgical access options, arthrodesis surgery introduces additional possible complications. When a bone fusion between two vertebrae is aimed for, but the bone does not heal properly, this leads to an abnormal joint. Movement- or loading-induced pain may be the end result.

However, as long as the osteosynthesis hardware provides stability, this should not be a problem. The problem arises when screws start to loosen. An adverse reflex sometimes seen is that the surgeon replaces the screws with thicker screws, or that the surgeon removes the screws (believing that the screws are the problem). When screws loosen, it either means that the mechanical construct is not sound (disequilibrium between loads and load-bearing capacities because of weak bone, alignment problems, etc.) and should be thought through again, or that there is a low grade infection at hand. Anyhow, situations with non-union and loosened screws may be a possible cause of pain. Still, diagnosing it as the true cause of pain is not easy, and rates of successful axial pain reduction by redo surgery are as low as 40-50 percent.

Another complication, already pointed to in the chapters on cervical spine surgery, is the phenomenon of adjacent level disease, which holds true for the lumbar spine as well. Fused segments behave as a lever arm that will increase loads and intradiscal pressure in the adjacent discs, accelerating degeneration and potentially resulting in symptomatic canal narrowing possibly associated with antero- or (more often) retrolisthesis. There is also an association between the occurrence of upper level adjacent level problems and insufficient lordosis at the fused segment. This brings us to a next possible complication. When two or more vertebrae are fused in a relative position of which the lordotic angles are lower than they should be to have the patient's centre of gravity above the sacrum, the patient will have to rely on overstretching the above levels and on heavy muscular effort to stand and walk in balance. Techniques exist to calculate the desired lordotic angle over a construct to fit the patient's individual spinopelvic anatomy and alignment. A violation of the sagittal balance principles leads to the so-called 'flat back' syndrome, in which the patient develops severe muscular pain when being upright for more than 10-15 minutes.

Finally, adding arthrodesis to a surgical action makes the surgery more invasive: longer muscle retraction, more risk of surgical manipulation and inadvertent damage of ligaments, facet capsule tissue and other structures that contribute to the complex interplay essential for optimal postural control. The more aggressive the surgery is, the higher the risk that postural control may be impaired. With each redo surgical action at a certain level, the chances of a satisfying outcome gradually decrease. All these factors together contribute to what is commonly referred to as 'failed back surgery syndrome'. Many surgeons feel this terminology puts blame on them, while the patient's situation is due to failure of a larger multidisciplinary context. Therefore, currently, the term 'failed back management syndrome' has been introduced. While these terms reflect a certain lack of ambition to better understand and manage the degenerative spinal problems, the existence of 'failed management' is unfortunately a reality.

Surprisingly and interestingly, no association ever has been demonstrated in literature between the actual achievement of bone fusion and patient functional outcomes.

6. LUMBAR STENOSIS IN DEFORMITY

Lumbar stenosis without deformity is described in chapter 4, including symptoms and management. In this chapter, the effect of two types of deformity on stenosis will be described separately, because it can affect management. Symptoms and differential diagnosis will not be repeated here.

Spondylolisthesis refers to the forward (antero-) or backward (retro-) slippage of the above vertebral body with respect to the lower one. In the lower spine, usually anterolisthesis is encountered, whereas retrolisthesis is more often seen in the upper lumbar spine. Spondylolisthesis may result from trauma, earlier surgery or bone tumour, but the most frequent etiologies are degenerative, spondylolysis and facet joint dysplasia. Degenerative anterolisthesis results from reduced disc height and facet joint capsule laxity, sometimes in combination with a tendency to sagittal remodelling of the facet joint gaps. Degenerative anterolisthesis usually occurs at L4L5, sometimes at L3L4, and has a high prevalence in the older population, particularly in females. As this is a type of degeneration, associated yellow ligament thickening and facet hypertrophy may cause central and/or lateral recess stenosis. Also the foramen may be narrowed. Typical of an anterolisthetic anatomy is that the nerve root will be trapped in between the pedicle and the pseudodisc bulging (i.e. the disc bridging the anteroposterior distance of the anterolisthesis which makes it look as if it bulges). In other words, the nerve root will be compressed in a craniocaudal direction.

A similar phenomenon is seen in anterolisthesis secondary to bilateral spondylolysis. Spondylolysis refers to the lysis of the isthmus (also called isthmolysis), which usually is initiated as a stress fracture at adolescent age (most frequent in athletes) that fails to heal. Bilateral spondylolysis, most often seen at L5, may lead to a certain degree of anterolisthesis, which will remain asymptomatic. However, when the disc dehydrates and loses height at older age, anterolisthesis may increase and the foramen will be deformed as described above, leading to uni- or bilateral radicular pain from foraminal nerve root compression. In dysplastic spondylolisthesis, always at L5S1, patients have a congenital steep sacral slope in combination with dysplastic L5S1 facet joints that are unable to withhold gravity forces, resulting in anterior slippage of L5. Dysplastic spondylolisthesis may lead to severe degrees of L5S1 anterolisthesis. Radicular pain may result from traction on the L5 roots, as well as from foraminal stenosis and nerve root compression as described above.

A facet joint resection takes away the posterior wall of the foramen, but does not relieve the craniocaudal root compression. Therefore, in anterolisthetic foraminal stenosis, restoring disc height by means of an interbody cage is required for adequate nerve root decompression, at the same time making sure that the segmental lordotic angle is not reduced. In situations of central or lateral recess stenosis without foraminal stenosis in degenerative anterolisthesis (but not in lytic or dysplastic types), it has been demonstrated that simple interlaminar decompression without arthrodesis is sufficient in grade 1 anterolisthesis and provided the anterolisthesis is not unstable.

Degenerative scoliosis is associated with a lumbar scoliotic curve, usually dextroconvex and typically with its apex at or close to the L3 vertebra. At the concave side of the scoliotic curve, foraminal height is reduced, potentially resulting in craniocaudal nerve root compression and radicular pain (hence, usually L3). A concavity also exists where the lumbar spine meets the sacrum (called the 'fractional curve'), potentially resulting in L5 compression in the L5S1 foramen, and this is more often a problem than the midlumbar reduced foraminal height. Simple foraminal decompression may sometimes offer temporary relief of radicular pain, but in case of Cobb angle differences between standing and lying position or presence of laterolisthesis, simple decompression is not advocated. At the same time, this means that tackling the radicular compression will need to be associated with elaborate arthrodesis surgery taking care of the coronal and sagittal curves.

7. THORACOLUMBAR DEFORMITY

Adult spinal deformity refers to inadequate alignment of the thoracolumbar spine in the coronal and sagittal planes that pushes the patient outside his cone of efficient and optimal muscular energy use for maintaining posture during standing and walking. It represents a debilitating cause of axial pain and functional decline, and may manifest as scoliosis, thoracic hyperkyphosis or insufficient lumbar lordosis. The etiology is degenerative, with either de novo deformity or degenerative worsening of adolescent idiopathic scoliosis, but also sometimes iatrogenic (following lumbar arthrodesis surgery, see chapter 5). Surgical techniques have been developed to correct spinal curves by osteotomies and subsequent arthrodesis, that should be carefully planned and prepared, and performed in experienced hands and under neuromonitoring. Re-balancing the spine may have spectacular effects on the patient's functioning, but complication rates are in keeping with the invasiveness of the surgery, and later additional surgery is often required. Therefore, the quality of counselling is crucial. Patients should be well informed by experts, and pros and cons should be carefully weighted, taking into account comorbidities, frailty and expectations.

8. OTHER THAN TRAUMATIC AND DEGENERATIVE CONDITIONS

As stated in previous chapters, the physiotherapist should be able to detect and appropriately refer red flag conditions (see chapter 11). Red flag situations may lead to surgery and require postoperative physiotherapy.

Tumours and infections can occur in the lumbosacral spine, as they do in the cervical and thoracic spine, and I refer to chapter 5 of the cervical and thoracic spine text respectively for more extensive explanation. Patients with spinal metastasis and unstable pathological fractures and/or significant conus or cauda equina compression are candidates for surgical stabilisation or debulking and stabilisation, followed by radiotherapy. Primary malignant bone tumours can also occur in the lumbosacral spine. En bloc spondylectomy is technically feasible in the lumbar spine, but will inevitably be associated with sacrifice of nerve roots and subsequent neurological deficit. This also holds true in the sacral spine, which is a predilection site for chordomas, and the cranial extension will determine what nerve roots are required to be sacrificed for en bloc resection, and hence, the magnitude of postoperative motor and sphincter sequelae. Reduction of recurrence risk will have to be weighted against functional sequelae, also taking into account expected effects of other treatment modalities such as (proton) radiation and chemotherapy.

Infections causing instability require pedicle screw fixation. When neurological deficits arise from epidural abscess compressing the conus and/or cauda equina, decompression by laminectomy or by corpectomy and reconstruction should be performed. Source control by resection of the infectious mass and spinal reconstruction is only required in patients that are septic and are not responding to targeted antibiotic treatment. Following accurate debridement and under targeted antibiotics, instrumentation hardware can be safely used, even in infection cases.

Deformity conditions, described in the previous chapter, require specific expertise regarding evolution and operative possibilities and patients are eligible for expert advice from an orthopaedic department with experience in spinal deformity surgery.

9. POSTOPERATIVE REHABILITATION

Most of the evidence on postoperative rehabilitation available in literature deals with the lumbar spine. Postoperative rehabilitation has been shown to be safe, both in decompression as in arthrodesis surgery, also when started as early as 2 weeks after surgery. Some studies advocate multimodality rehabilitation to be superior over exercising alone. However, reported beneficial effects are usually short term, and most studies fail to unequivocally prove long-term benefit. On the other hand, this may not be surprising, given the heterogeneity of the patient population and the ongoing dynamics of degeneration. Acknowledging the immense effect of patients' beliefs, worries and attitudes, it is my experience and opinion that accurate guidance and coaching is of utmost importance in the peri- and postoperative period, and well-trained physiotherapists play a huge role. From experience, we have learnt that preoperative group or individual physiotherapy sessions have an enormous impact on reducing immediately postoperative anxieties, and that early and physiotherapy-guided mobilisation sets the stage for patients' trust in further activities. Before starting more intensive physiotherapy after discharge from the hospital, a short period (1-2 weeks) of soft tissue healing is best taken into account, after which physiotherapy will focus on education, optimising further soft tissue healing, managing misbalance and dysfunction and gradual reconditioning to be fit for desired participation.

Interestingly, the attitude towards rehabilitation following arthrodesis surgery should in fact not be different from decompression surgery. No fusion surgeries without insertion of osteosynthesis hardware are being done any more. Hence, a well-performed arthrodesis is stable and secure enough, and the physiotherapist will not 'break the screws'. In reality, however, actual practice will usually depend on logistic issues and surgeons' beliefs and habits. The patient should never wear a brace in the postoperative period. There is no evidence that supports postoperative braces, and in fact they do more harm to the mind of the patient than they do anything else. The only exception to the latter (for the lumbar spine) are the patients with a conservatively treated fracture. Even there, however, no hard evidence on braces exists, and they are predominantly being used in young and active patients, rather than in osteoporotic fractures. In the conservatively treated trauma population, physiotherapy is also helpful: in the older population to stimulate self-care and ADL; in the younger patients to start reconditioning stabilisers before the brace is removed.

Return to work is an important issue. Long-term absence from work – because of pain and disability in the preoperative period and because of anxieties and mixed messages from both caregivers and employers ('you should be properly recovered') – is a disease on its own. When a patient fails to go back to work within 6 months, chances of eventually getting back to work become grim. All caregivers (including the occupational physicians) should stimulate the patient to resume work as soon as possible. This requires good communication between all partners, proactive policies and emphasis on individual work hardening strategies.

10. WHAT ABOUT AXIAL PAIN?

According to evidence and international guidelines, no surgery should be performed in axial low back pain. Arthrodesis and disc prosthesis surgery lead to unpredictable results, often better indeed in the short term of months following surgery, and then getting worse in the longer run. A main reason for this phenomenon is that the contribution to outcome variability of psychosocial risk factors is much larger than the contribution of the type and quality of surgery. This holds true for so-called 'degenerative disc disease', as well as for spondylolisthesis or other deformities. The answer on how these patients should be addressed is found in the overall triage concept outlined in the introduction of this book. Red flags should be ruled out first, then radicular pain should be looked for and the management of axial pain depends on the timeline: the further a patient proceeds in time, the more should be invested in addressing psychosocial risk factors and in incremental rehabilitation efforts to avoid chronicity.

In chronic low back pain, rehabilitation potential and all relevant risk factors should be carefully assessed, and in my opinion specialists in physical medicine are in the best position for this. As stated, in principle surgery should not be performed. However, in medicine, nothing is really black or white. Some very selective situations exist in which surgery can potentially be considered. The Belgian low back pain pathway indicates that the physical medicine specialist can turn to the surgeon in the multi/interdisciplinary spine clinic to discuss these. Examples are the unstable spondylolisthesis, postsurgical instability, non-union or adjacent level disease. In case of deformity and persistent problems, it may be useful to ask for an expert orthopaedic surgery consult. In such situations, all relevant patient-related factors should be taken into account and surgery will be embedded in a multidisciplinary trajectory.

11. RED FLAGS IN THE LUMBOSACRAL SPINE

CAUDA EQUINA SYNDROME	• Preceding intense low back pain • Saddle (perianal, perineal) numbness or tingling • Sphincter disturbances: usually urinary retention and obstipation, but potentially loss of sphincter control (urinary incontinence, faecal or flatus incontinence, lax anal sphincter at palpation) • Sexual dysfunction • Uni- or bilateral radicular pain • Severe or progressive neurological deficits in the lower limbs (L5, S1, S2) and/or gait difficulties

RUPTURED AORTA ANEURYSM	• Man > 50 years with vascular risk factors: smoking, arterial hypertension, hyper-cholesterolemia, diabetes mellitus … • Intense pain in the back as well as in the abdomen, often radiation in the L3 dermatome is reported • Unwell, shock • Pulsating abdominal mass
TRAUMATIC FRACTURE	• Sudden onset of pain and possibility of traumatic event • New onset structural spinal deformity • Severe pain, pain better when lying down • Known or suspected ankylosing spondylitis or DISH and onset of back pain following (even minor) trauma (= fracture until otherwise proven)
INFECTIOUS DISORDER	• Severe and continuous low back pain • Pain worse at night, pain that is not affected by position or movement • Fever, chills • Recent gastro-intestinal/gynaecological infection or surgery • Recent lumbar spine surgery • Immune suppression • Intravenous drug use • Recent bacterial infection • Older age

SPINAL TUMOUR	• New onset low back pain in a patient older than 50 years (55 years in some guidelines) or younger than 20 years • History of cancer • Persistent pain, pain worse at night, pain that is not affected by position or movement • New onset structural spinal deformity • Pain in different locations • Unexplained weight loss
OSTEOPOROTIC COMPRESSION FRACTURE	• Sudden onset axial pain after a brisk movement or (even minor) trauma in patient known or suspected with osteoporosis or long-term steroid use • New onset structural spinal deformity • Severe pain, pain better when lying down
INFLAMMATORY PAIN	• Young adult • Morning stiffness • Pain at rest, less pain during movement • Pain at night, particularly in the second half of the night • Pain when tired • Swinging gluteal pains • History of auto-immune disease in the patient or a first-grade relative (eg. m. Crohn's, colitis ulcerosa, uveitis, Graves')

| **NEFROLITHIASIS CRISIS (RENAL COLIC)** | • Intense, almost intolerable cramp-like pain in the upper lumbar spine region radiating to the groin and genital areas
• Burning sensation and pain during micturition
• Nausea and vomiting
• Intense pain when tapping on the paramedian spinal region at the level of the kidney
• Red blood in urine |

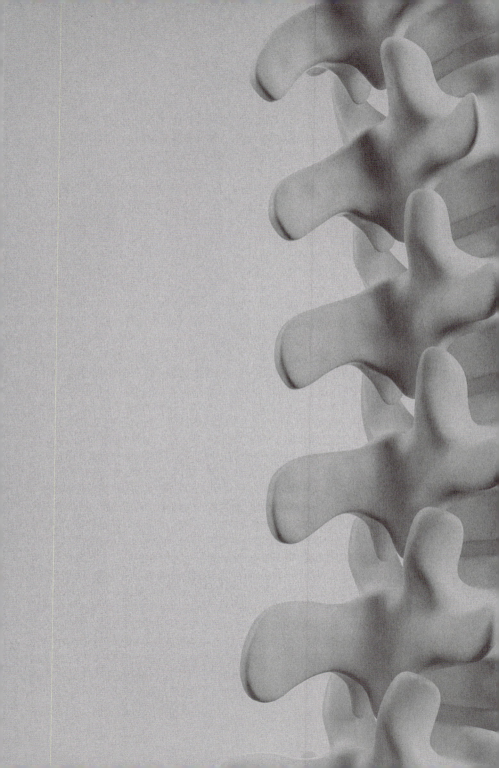

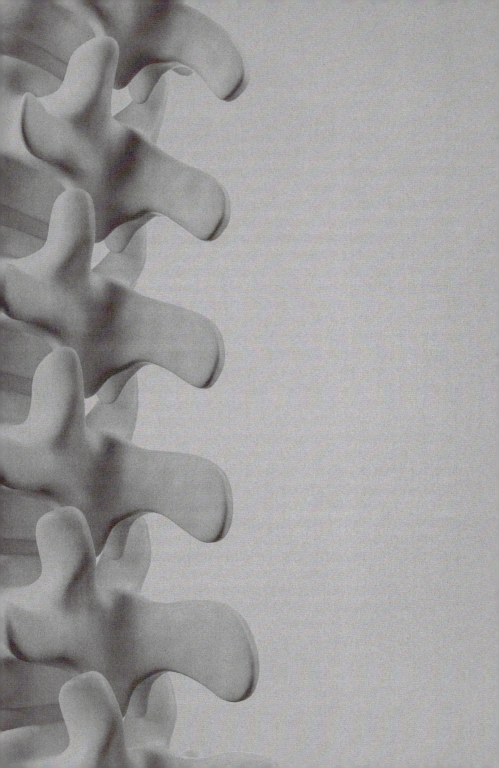

VOCABULARY OF SURGICAL PROCEDURES

Corpectomy
The removal of (a large part of) a vertebral body including the disc above and below. This is usually done from an anterior approach (cervical, thoracic, lumbar), but may also be done posteriorly in the thoracic spine. The body is removed in pieces (piecemeal resection), and a reconstruction by a cage will be necessary.

Costotransversectomy
The removal in the thoracic spine of the medial part of the rib, the transverse process and the pedicle in order to establish a lateral view on the thecal sac and posterior part of the thoracic vertebral body. This is sometimes performed in soft thoracic disc herniation surgery, or to make an entry to a tumour in the vertebral body.

Discectomy
In anterior surgery, both in the cervical and lumbar spine, a discectomy refers to the removal of the entire disc, including annulus fibrosus and nucleus pulposus, including the cleaning of the upper and lower endplates, and will require reconstruction by a cage. However, in posterior lumbar surgery, the term discectomy is used for the emptying of the nucleus pulposus in disc herniation surgery through the original defect in the posterior annulus fibrosus, in which the rest of the annulus stays untouched. When this is done under the microscope, people call it a 'microdiscectomy'. When a disc herniation is removed without manipulating the nucleus pulposus, usually people nowadays use the term 'sequestromy', see below.

Facetectomy

Facetectomy refers to the removal of an entire facet joint. This may be needed to drastically open up the foramen in a foraminal stenosis in the lumbar spine, or to make an approach for a TLIF (see below) or (done bilaterally) to create the possibility to increase lordosis in deformity surgery. After a facetectomy, arthrodesis of that motion level is required.

Foraminotomy

When a narrow foramen is made a bit larger, this is called a foraminotomy. This usually concerns the medial aspect of the foramen by an intraspinal route but sometimes also the lateral aspect of the foramen by an extraforaminal approach. The isthmus should not be damaged because segmental instability would result.

Fusion

Fusion refers to the bone healing resulting in two bones (two vertebrae) fusing together. As the fusion is nowadays always facilitated by using osteosynthesis hardware to ensure immediate stability, the term 'fusion' is often used as a pars pro toto referring to the entire procedure. However, strictly speaking, the 'fusion' part of a surgery, and the instrumentation (the placing of osteosynthesis hardware) are two different things. Therefore in this book, the generic term 'arthrodesis' will be used. This allows us to reserve the term 'fusion' for the procedure that aims at achieving bone fusion, and for the process of bone fusion itself.

ACIF

Anterior Cervical Interbody Fusion, meaning that a cage with bone or bone substitute is placed in the intervertebral space following discectomy through an anterior approach. This is possible from C2C3 to C7T1.

ALIF

Anterior Lumbar Interbody Fusion, meaning that a cage with bone or bone substitute is placed in the intervertebral space following discectomy through an anterior abdominal (retroperitoneal) approach. This is possible at L4L5 and L5S1.

DLIF

Direct Lateral Interbody Fusion, meaning that a cage with bone or bone substitute is placed in the lumbar intervertebral space following discectomy through a lateral retroperitoneal transpsoas approach. This is done at L1L2 to L4L5.

OLIF

Oblique Lumbar Interbody Fusion, meaning that a cage with bone or bone substitute is placed in the intervertebral space following discectomy through an oblique anterior abdominal (retroperitoneal) approach. This is done at L1L2 to L4L5.

PLIF

Posterior Lumbar Interbody Fusion, meaning that two cages with bone or bone substitute are placed in the intervertebral space following discectomy (nucleus pulposus and endplate cartilage) through a posterior interlaminar approach, for each cage (right and left) by removing the inferior articular process of the upper level and retracting the thecal sac medially.

PLF

Posterior Lumbar Fusion, meaning that bone grafts are placed in the gutter formed by the lateral facet joints and transverse processes. Also the 'facet fusions' in which the facet joint gap is drilled and bone grafts are put in the joint gap are being called posterior fusions.

TLIF

Transforaminal Lumbar Interbody Fusion, meaning that a cage with bone or bone substitute is placed in the intervertebral space following discectomy (nucleus pulposus and endplate cartilage) through the foraminal area of the disc, i.e. in between the exiting nerve root of that level and the shoulder of the lower nerve root, which requires the resection of the entire facet joint at one side. The cage is then inserted in such a way that it crosses the midline, or multiple cages are inserted.

XLIF

The Extreme Lateral Interbody Fusion is a synonym for DLIF.

Interlaminar decompression

The removal of yellow ligament in between two laminae, keeping the laminae, facet joints and midline (spinous processes and inter/supraspinous ligaments) intact. This is performed to decompress the thecal sac in case of yellow ligament hypertrophy.

Laminectomy

The removal of an entire lamina, including its spinous process and the yellow ligament above and below it. Not advocated for decompression in the lumbar spine anymore, because the interlaminar decompression fits that purpose perfectly. Still sometimes performed in the cervical and thoracic spine. A laminectomy is sometimes preferred when a larger exposure of the thecal sac is required, eg. to remove an extradural or intradural tumour.

Laminotomy

Literally this means the cutting of a lamina with a high speed laminotome. This is done in intradural tumour surgery, after which the lamina is placed back and fixated with small screws and plates or wire. In the English literature, the term 'laminotomy' is also used to refer to an interlaminar decompression.

Laminoplasty

In a laminoplasty or 'open door laminoplasty', the cervical lamina is cut at one side and thinned on the other side, and then opened towards the side of the thinning, which acts as a hinge by creating a greenstick fracture. On the other side, the lamina is kept open by a small piece of metal or bone. This is done to enlarge the cervical spinal canal in degenerative cervical myelopathy. It has the advantage of installing a barrier between the thecal sac and muscles and maintains mobility.

Sequestrectomy

Removing only the herniated nucleus pulposus, keeping the inside of the disc untouched, is called a sequestrectomy. It is done in the lumbar spine, and also in the cervical spine when the surgeon decides that the hernia is lateral enough to the thecal sac (with the spinal cord) to safely remove it from the back.

Spondylectomy

The term 'spondylectomy' or 'en bloc spondylectomy' refers to the radical removal in one piece of a vertebra containing a tumour (as opposed to piecemeal resections). When the lamina is tumour free and can be opened without breaching the tumour, the rest of the vertebra can be detached from its surroundings and gently be pushed away from the thecal sac, obviously requiring stabilisation during and following the procedure. This can be done in the thoracic and lumbar spine, but is only required in some malignant primary bone tumours.

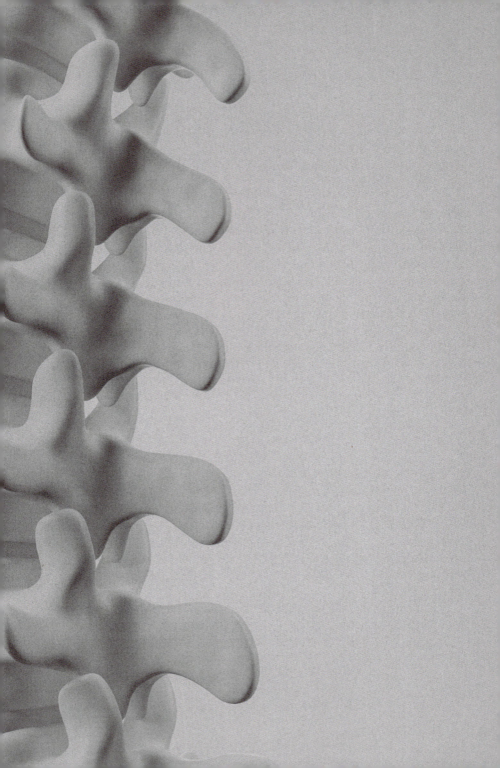

ADL	activities of daily life
CT	computed tomography
DISH	diffuse idiopathic skeletal hyperostosis
MRC	Medical Research Council
MRI	magnetic resonance imaging
PEEK	polyether ether ketone

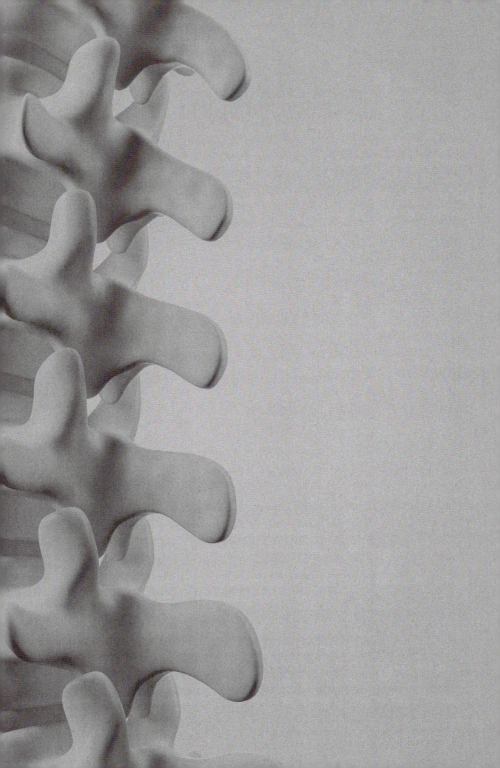

ACKNOWLEDGEMENTS

I wish to thank Dr Thomas Decramer, neurosurgeon, and MSc. Ann Spriet, for their willingness to read the manuscript and provide me with their extremely helpful advice.

I dedicate this work to all my loved ones.

Quality is never an accident. It is always the result of high intention, sincere effort, intelligent direction and skilful execution. It represents the wise choice of many alternatives, the cumulative experience of many masters of craftsmanship.

William A. Foster

D/2021/45/590 – NUR 877, 892
ISBN 978 94 014 8254 7

COVER DESIGN   Adept vormgeving
PAGE DESIGN   Keppie & Keppie

© Bart Depreitere & Lannoo Publishers nv, Tielt, 2022.

LannooCampus Publishers is a subsidiary of Lannoo Publishers,
the book and multimedia division of Lannoo Publishers nv.

LannooCampus Publishers
Vaartkom 41 box 01.02
3001 Leuven
Belgium
WWW.LANNOOCAMPUS.COM

P.O. BOX 23202
1100 DS Amsterdam
Netherlands